Fun on Foot in New York

Warwick Ford

with Nola Ford

Wyltan Books
Aspen, Colorado, U.S.A.

This book is designed to help you make decisions regarding your fitness program and training. It is not intended as a substitute for professional fitness and medical advice. As with all fitness programs, you should seek your doctor's approval before you begin.

There are safety risks inherent in running, jogging, and walking. Neither the publisher nor authors shall be liable for injury or harm allegedly resulting from reading this book. The publisher and authors make no representations or warranties, express or implied, and hereby disclaim the implied warranties of merchantability or fitness for a particular purpose, with respect to this book or any sales and marketing materials promoting this book.

Wyltan and Fun on Foot are trademarks of Wyltan, Inc.

ISBN 978-0-9765244-2-7   paperback
ISBN-10: 0-9765244-2-2   paperback
Library of Congress Control Number: 2008923506

Printed in the United States of America by BookMasters, Inc.
Front cover photo: The authors in Central Park, New York.
Back cover photo: ING New York City Marathon finish, photograph courtesy of New York Road Runners. Used with permission.
Geographical and street information in maps courtesy the U.S. Geological Survey.

Available in bookstores and online at http://www.funonfoot.com.

Wyltan Books
Aspen, Colorado, U.S.A.
http://www.funonfoot.com

This is a 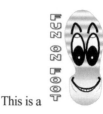 Book

Table of Contents

Preface

For many years I have known that outdoor exercise—running, jogging, or walking—can greatly boost life's enjoyment and longevity. However, I also know that that understanding does not always translate successfully into actually spending more time outdoors exercising. In my case, the most challenging period was when I worked as a Silicon Valley executive and was continually on the road, visiting different U.S. cities. I found it very difficult to motivate myself to go for a run in an unfamiliar place—too many things might conceivably go wrong.

I realized I would run more if I had a book telling me what to expect outdoors in a city, and suggesting some really good places to go for exercise. Since no such book existed, I started doing my own research and taking copious notes. That led eventually, with the collaboration of my charming wife Nola, to the publication of *Fun on Foot in America's Cities*. That title was targeted primarily at the frequent traveler who visits different cities and can use some help and motivation to get outdoors and run, jog, or walk. The main idea was to arm the reader with the information needed to quickly locate comfortable and enjoyable on-foot routes in our largest cities.

Fun on Foot in America's Cities is particularly popular with travelers, ranging from serious marathon runners through to people who just walk long distances regularly. However, that title is of less value to people who usually stay near home. Such people want information and ideas about their own region rather than places they never visit. We therefore decided to produce regionally focused adaptations of the Fun-on-Foot model for the cities we know well. We started with *Fun on Foot in New England*, focusing on the Boston region and other New England centers.

Now we come to *Fun on Foot in New York*, focusing on New York City and its surroundings. This is definitely our most exciting work, being about the world's most exciting city, and a place where we have been running and exploring for many years.

In this latest title, we give more attention than in earlier titles to competitive running events in the places covered. Both Nola and I are becoming increasingly involved in road racing. While I am not so young, not fast, and do not expect to ever win a race, I greatly enjoy participating in community races. The anticipation of a future race also helps me get out more and work harder. Nevertheless, this book's target audience is not limited to competitive runners.

Nola and I have also become increasingly involved in various running clubs and realize how helpful they can be to local residents, newcomers, and visitors to an area. Consequently, in this book we include information to help link up our readers with running clubs in their locality of interest.

The information we provide on individual clubs has been paraphrased from statements provided by club representatives or extracted (with permission) from club websites. Therefore, we do not claim originality of this material nor can we take responsibility for its accuracy.

This book is supported by the website www.funonfoot.com, which will publish up-to-the-minute information for the New York runner or walker, updates to book content, and links to other on-line resources useful to the reader. Please visit this site for that information and for an opportunity to share your own ideas and opinions with the Fun-on-Foot community. We shall also be distributing from that site, for a nominal charge, a downloadable printer-friendly compilation of all maps in this book.

* * * *

Many people contributed in various ways to the compilation and production of this book. We particularly want to thank the following local athletes for major contributions or critical reviews of material about their own turf: Russ Charlton (Manhattan); Brad Skillman and Dave Mendelsohn (Brooklyn); Bonnie Harper and Jared Mestre (Queens); Bob Beattie (Long Island); and Mike Barnow (Westchester).

From the many running clubs we communicated with, we want to particularly thank two clubs that hosted us personally in their activities and so helped us greatly in accumulating ideas. The first is the Prospect

Park Track Club, where we want to especially thank Gil Torres, Wayne Bailey, Al Prawda and Zoe, Tyrone Sklaren, Geoff Vincent, and Cecil Burgin. The other club is the Alley Pond Striders, where we want to acknowledge Howard Cohen, Herb Ascher, Ray Dowe, and Jerry Ruiz.

We also want to thank New York Road Runners for their help and support in various ways.

The following individuals also stand out for their special help in researching this project or reviewing the manuscript: Michael Balbos; Jack Biggane; John Boykin; Laura Clark; Leigh Cohen; Pete Colaizzo; Ray Constantino; Lyall Ford; Brian Foster; Harry Greco; Fred Haslett; Joe Hornyak; Ed McLaughlin; Mary Molski; Greg Mulligan; Jeanne Paliswiat; Karen Randall; Dorothy Reilly; Ken Rolston; Barbara Rushman; Robin Schiffman; Lorrie Tily; Deirdre Venables; and Noel Weil.

Thank you all for your contributions and for sharing with us your knowledge of your part of the New York region.

Thanks also to the folk at BookMasters for their ever-reliable production work.

Nola and I hope you will enjoy reading and using this book, and that it contributes in some little way to your future quality of life.

Warwick Ford

• • • • • • • • • •	**Featured on-foot route**
· · · · · · · · · · ·	**Other on-foot routes**
- - - - - - - -	**Rail track**
- · - · - · - · ·	**State or county boundary**
————————	**Street**
— — — —	**Major highway (No pedestrians)**
🚆	**Train station**
🚌	**Bus stop**
⛴	**Ferry dock**
Ⓜ	**NYC subway station**
🚻	**Restroom (Year-round)**
🚻	**Restroom (Seasonal or portable)**
🚰	**Drinking water (Possibly seasonal)**
🍴	**Eating/drinking establishment**
🅿	**Trail parking**
①	**Point of interest**

Key to Map Symbols

1

Introduction

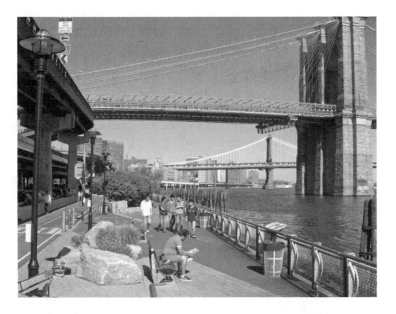

N ew York City and its surrounds are a delight for those of us who like to get outdoors to run, jog, or walk. Thanks to the extensive coastline and rivers, and to the generous park and trail systems, there are many excellent places to exercise on-foot. A good public transit system helps us get around the region, opening up a variety of options for places to run on different days. However, because of the massive road traffic volumes and the crowding of people in certain places, not all on-foot routes are equal. They range from outstanding in quality and pleasantness to noisy, ugly, and dull. A goal of this book is to spell out the respective qualities of different routes, removing the uncertainties for runners and walkers.[1]

1   Chapter head photo: The East River trail in Lower Manhattan.

We do not limit our coverage to just the city. We extend it to a number of population centers throughout New York State and New Jersey that have good running and walking trails nearby.

If you are a runner, jogger, or athletic walker and either visit this region or are moving to live here, we believe you will find this book invaluable. If you already live in this region, and are seeking ideas to make your runs or walks more interesting or to motivate you to get out more, this book is also for you.

Whether you are a committed athlete in training, an occasional jogger, or someone struggling to gain fitness and lose weight, you will appreciate this book. It will help to remove the barriers to your spending more time outdoors and building fitness while enjoying the region.

Motivation

If you feel you sometimes lack motivation to get outdoors on foot, read this section. (Committed athletes can skip to the next section.)

One of the easiest and most effective ways to keep fit and control weight is to run, jog, or walk in attractive, comfortable, and interesting environments. There are too many excuses for skipping exercise, which is frequently considered a chore, if not downright unpleasant. Exercise must be easy and enjoyable if we are to regularly get off our butts.

On-foot exercise—running, jogging, or walking—is an excellent way to keep fit, but doing it in a gym does not pass the ease and enjoyment test (not to mention the budget test) with many people. *Outdoor* on-foot exercise, on the other hand, can definitely be easy and enjoyable. However, one is often unsure of where to go and what to expect on the way. Many people hesitate to head out on a new route they do not know intimately. All too often, this leads to a convenient excuse for staying indoors or in-vehicle. We help you get out on foot by leading you to the very best outdoor exercise routes in your region of interest.

My wife and running partner, Nola, and I have both suffered at times from a lack of motivation to get out running. However, since taking the approach of always seeking new, attractive, and interesting places to run, we have kept the motivation alive and succeeded in keeping fit.

Our Fun-on-Foot books do not generally distinguish between running, jogging, and walking as forms of exercise. While faster exercise builds fitness and burns calories more quickly, all forms are good. Before Nola and I started serious training, on a typical outing we always started out jogging. If either of our bodies started to protest loudly enough along the way, we would fall back to walking later. However, we always finished the route. We believe that is most important.

One thing that surprises me is the number of people who are reluctant to try our routes saying, "I can't walk three miles, and certainly not ten!" When pressed to try, they usually retract those preconceptions. Almost anyone without serious disabilities can walk three miles without pain in under an hour and ten miles in three hours or so.

If you are prepared to do some walking but cannot or will not run or jog, this book is still for you. You might be surprised at how rapidly your distances and times improve.

When I say walking, I mean walking at a good pace—not strolling. One of the main impediments we on-foot exercisers face is the person who strolls along at a snail's pace, blocking the sidewalk or pedestrian trail and making no attempt to get his or her blood pumping.

While slow pedestrians are a pain, there is one other entity that really is our Public Enemy Number 1: the *automobile*. The more we can tame our urge to get into that metal box, the more walking, jogging, or running we shall inevitably do. Therefore, we try to exclude or minimize automobile dependence throughout our travels in the Fun-on-Foot books.

Where to Go?

When seeking information or ideas on running routes in any locality, there is ample commentary to be found on websites, in local publications, or from your friendly hotel concierge or visitor information booth. However, in my experience, that information too often proves to be sketchy, out-of-date, rose-tinted, or otherwise unreliable or inaccurate. Nola and I continue to be surprised at how frequently the ideas from these sources leave us disappointed when we follow them up in practice.

That is why this book is needed. We always try to be objective. We have a well-defined model for assessing routes and we endeavor to apply a consistent standard everywhere.

For every region covered, we try to find the very best outdoor exercise routes and describe them in detail as *featured routes*. We mainly seek routes in the three-to-ten mile range—distances that are not too long for a half-day walk and long enough for a nice run for all but the serious distance runner. In some cases you can link up multiple routes to increase the distance substantially.

Routes are assessed in terms of four attributes: (1) comfort; (2) attractions; (3) convenience; and (4) a destination.

Comfort, which is the most essential attribute, has several elements. First, there should be minimal safety concerns. There should be a reasonable expectation that there will not be a nasty surprise around the next corner.[1] The number of other people around should be in your comfort zone (not too many and not too few). Underfoot conditions should also be good and there should be a minimum of encounters with vehicular traffic.

Attractions are what make a route environmentally pleasant and interesting. It helps enormously if a route has points of historic or cultural interest, scenic beauty, or people activities on the day. To be interesting, variety is also desirable. Any route can become boring with time, so it is good to have some elements to vary each time. Also, we prefer to avoid out-and-back routes. Repeating everything you saw in the first half of a route on the way back can be less satisfying than having something new to see all the way. Therefore, we try to create loop routes or find ways to return to the start of a one-way route using another form of transportation.

Convenience means ease of getting to the start of a route from a nearby population center or areas where visitors tend to stay. Similarly, getting back from the end of a route should be easy. Given our belief that the number one enemy of on-foot fitness is the automobile, we try to avoid the need for automobiles in getting to, from, or along our routes. If other forms of transportation are required to close a loop, we look mainly to public transit, so as to minimize costs, hassle, and automobile dependence.

Destination is an important factor for some people. Serious runners frequently gain their on-foot satisfaction from successfully meeting their own time and distance goals, and are then content to get straight back to their home or hotel for a shower. However, many people struggle to get out on foot and to complete a route of sufficient distance. Having a clear destination in mind helps make a route motivating

---

1   See the subsequent section on "Are These Routes Safe?".

and also reduces the temptation to quit early. If you are mentally on a mission to go somewhere enjoyable, then odds are you will make it there. Therefore, we consider it valuable for routes to finish in places where there is something interesting to see or do afterwards.

One aspect of a destination that helps many people is having a good food/beverage break available at the end. Nola and I have found this works for us. When we first started pushing ourselves to run more, it became apparent that Nola was way more likely to start and complete an eight-mile weekend jog if there was a tasty brunch at the end. I was way more likely to do the same if there was a glass of cold beer where we finished.

Consequently, one theme you will find in this book is the idea of ending routes near good eating and drinking establishments, where you can wind down if you so choose. We tend to look for pub-restaurants—informal places that will happily accept people in running gear and a little untidy.

Running, Walking, and Losing Weight

On-foot exercise burns many calories, with the following table giving a rough guide.[2]

Body Weight:	110 lb. (50 Kg.)	150 lb. (68 Kg.)	190 lb. (86 Kg.)
Walking 5 miles	380	500	650
Jogging 5 miles	392	530	674
Running 5 miles	432	567	708
Walking 10 miles	760	1,000	1,300
Jogging 10 miles	783	1,060	1,348
Running 10 miles	864	1,134	1,416

Estimated Calories Burned in a 5- or 10-mile Route
Assumed speeds: Walking 3.0 mph, Jogging 5.2 mph, Running 7.5 mph

2   Figures computed from data in: Maria Adams, MS, MPH, RD, "The Benefits and Risks of Walking Versus Running," HealthGate http://www. somersetmedicalcenter.com/110324.cfm. Note, however, that calorie burn rate depends on many factors including, but not limited to, amount of skeletal muscle, running efficiency, speed, surface type, incline, resting metabolism, level of fitness, and outside temperature. (Thanks to Ayesha Rollinson for explaining this.)

If you are concerned about using a food or beverage destination for motivation in completing an on-foot exercise excursion, be sure to take this factor into account.

Since we believe there is a correlation between the set of people who really relish a good meal or drink and the set of people who most need more exercise, we do not shy away from the food-and-drink motivation angle. A little extra indulgence in the food and drink department is a perfectly reasonable inducement to exercise, but only if you do the exercise first.

Why Not Just Follow the Bike Map?

New York City publishes an excellent, free bike map. Cycling is a fine fitness activity and we on-foot exercisers often share trails with cyclists, but choosing a good on-foot route can be very different to choosing a good cycling route.

In fact, we on-footers have many advantages over cyclists that allow us to find more interesting and attractive routes. Many places that are ideal for running or walking do not permit cycling or are just not suitable for cycling (think of steps, for example).

Especially when away from the home scene, the cyclist is faced with such problems as obtaining a bike, leaving it somewhere safe when going into a restaurant or shop, storing it in the evening, and getting it onto public transit (if that is even possible). On-footers face none of those problems.

We therefore decided not to limit our routes to paths suitable for cycling and, as a consequence, can frequently offer on-footers a superior experience.

Inline skating is closer to on-foot exercise. Some but not all of our routes are suitable for inline skating. In each route description, we try to assess the extent to which inline skating will work.

Are These Routes Safe?

Nola and I have personally checked out all the featured routes. We make a point of avoiding routes through areas where we feel uncomfortable—especially areas where we have observed questionable characters hanging about, where there are overt crime concerns, where there is a dearth of respectable outdoor exercisers, or where locals have warned us of risks.

However, this does not guarantee that you will not encounter trouble on our featured routes, or anywhere else. Always use good street-sense. On routes where other pedestrians are scarce, going with a partner is highly recommended. Even with such precautions, there is some residual risk of problems. The publisher and we authors disclaim all liability for problems encountered on the routes discussed in this book.

When in an unfamiliar place, a useful yardstick for safety expectations is its past record for violent crime as published by the FBI in its annual *Crime in the United States* report. To help you gain quick access to that report's data, we have distilled out a figure for violent crimes per head of population for various cities/towns in New York and New Jersey. The following tables list the number of reported violent crimes per 1,000 residents in 2006 (the latest year available at publication time). If concerned about safety, you might use extra caution in any place with an index over 10.[3]

New York City has a comparatively modest figure of 6.38, among the best for large U.S. cities. This provides us some reassurance that the Big Apple is not the dangerous place it once was. Certainly, I am amazed how safe it now feels in areas that I would not have ventured into alone 30 years ago.

On-Foot Conditions in New York City

Visitors or newcomers to New York City might find this section helpful. (City residents can skip to the next section.)

Running and jogging are popular in New York City, although they are largely limited to parks and trails along the rivers or the shore. In the high-density areas, including most of Manhattan, running through the streets can be questionable because of the many intersections encountered and the halts caused by the heavy vehicular and pedestrian traffic.

---

3   The FBI cautions against using its data for ranking communities and says: "Valid assessments are possible only with careful study and analysis of the range of unique conditions affecting each local law enforcement jurisdiction."

City/Town	Population in 2006	Violent Crimes per 1,000 Inhabitants
Albany	93,773	12.98
Amherst Town	112,284	1.09
Beacon	14,876	5.58
Binghamton	45,614	4.52
Buffalo	280,494	14.11
Cheektowaga Town	80,995	2.73
Clarkstown Town	78.642	0.84
Clay Town	54,356	0.29
Colonie Town	77,357	1.22
Dobbs Ferry Village	11,100	0.99
East Hampton Town	18,989	1.58
Greece Town	94,233	1.03
Hastings-on-Hudson	7,723	2.85
Hempstead Village	52,970	6.15
Hyde Park Town	20,922	0.05
Ithaca	29,846	2.08
Kingston	23,129	3.85
Mount Vernon	68,106	10.56
New Paltz	14,046	4.49
New Rochelle	73,162	3.31
New York	8,165,001	6.38
Newburgh	28,624	13.49
Niagara Falls	53,008	12.13
Poughkeepsie	30,436	13.70
Poughkeepsie Town	43,809	0.82
Ramapo Town	74,747	1.14
Rochester	211,656	12.60
Rome	34,436	1.31
Saratoga Springs	28,111	1.78
Schenectady	61,444	11.59
Southampton Town	50,311	1.57
Syracuse	142,062	10.66
Tonawanda Town	58,720	2.81
Troy	48,439	7.70
Utica	59,495	7.14
Watertown	27,293	6.52
White Plains	56,885	2.76
Yonkers	196,951	4.97

Violent Crime Rates for New York Cities in 2006
Source: FBI *Crime in the United States* Report 2006

City/Town	Population in 2006	Violent Crimes per 1,000 Inhabitants
Alpine	2,370	0.42
Asbury Park	16,637	23.20
Atlantic City	40,399	20.84
Bayonne	60,033	3.21
Belmar	5,967	5.87
Brick Twp	78,214	1.06
Camden	80,071	21.14
Cherry Hill Twp	71,876	1.49
Clifton	79,983	2.24
East Orange	68,242	10.54
Edison Twp	100,575	2.93
Elizabeth	125,905	7.10
Englewood	26,227	2.55
Fort Lee	37,203	0.51
Franklin Twp	58,505	1.50
Gloucester Twp	66,590	2.61
Hamilton Twp	90,062	2.31
Hoboken	39,930	2.88
Irvington	58,921	22.25
Jersey City	239,794	12.05
Lakewood Twp	68,886	3.27
Long Branch	32,115	5.36
Manasquan	6,206	0.64
Middletown Twp	67,877	0.84
Morristown	18,865	5.62
New Brunswick	50,194	7.17
Newark	280,877	10.11
Old Bridge Twp	64,903	0.83
Passaic	68,390	9.45
Paterson	149,957	11.15
Princeton	13,505	1.55
Sea Girt	2,071	2.90
Toms River Twp	94,732	1.18
Trenton	84,703	15.04
Union City	65,178	6.24
Ventnor City	12,747	1.41
Vineland	58,208	9.26
Woodbridge Twp	100,655	2.58

Violent Crime Rates for New Jersey Cities in 2006
Source: FBI *Crime in the United States* Report 2006

New York City's climate is very good for on-foot exercise. The average daily maximum is in the Fun-on-Foot preferred 40-to-80 degrees range every month except January, when it dips a little lower. There is precipitation on average 121 days of the year, so there is some risk of a shower dampening your day.

The biggest challenges that on-foot exercisers in New York City face relate to the massive road traffic volumes and the in-your-face vehicle presence almost everywhere.

New York City drivers are generally both very assertive and alert. That is the only way to survive as a driver in city traffic. Note, however, that many drivers give little consideration to pedestrians. This attitude is vastly different to that in many smaller centers and some other major cities. If you are crossing against a light in New York City, be prepared for vehicles to plough straight through a pedestrian crossing with the inevitable horn blast the only warning.

A big benefit for the on-foot exerciser in New York City is the ease of getting from almost anywhere to the best exercise routes, thanks to the excellent public transit system. The New York Subway system provides good coverage of Manhattan, Brooklyn, the Bronx, and some parts of Queens. Its frequency is generally good. The subway network is augmented by bus, ferry, and regional rail services. In our route descriptions we point out the public transit services near the start and finish points of the routes.

When necessary, you can always fall back to use of a taxi. The New York taxi system has been very good for many years, and the only recent complaint is that it is starting to get as pricey as other cities. This is always a reasonable transport option, especially in Manhattan.

There are many excellent restaurants and pubs throughout New York City that make for great food and beverage destinations. The dress codes that were once prevalent have largely gone out the window now, except for high-end restaurants. There is rarely a problem going into pubs or lower-end restaurants in running gear.

Running Clubs

Outdoor exercise becomes way easier if done in good company. Running with a personal buddy helps enormously.

Running clubs provide an opportunity for finding suitable running company and meeting local people who share an interest in a healthy lifestyle. Clubs can also provide access to coaching advice if you are interested in serious competition. New York City and the surrounding regions are blessed with a number of excellent running clubs, many being open to everyone, regardless of age, sex, race, speed, or running experience. While some clubs are highly competitive, in most the emphasis is more on encouragement to get out on foot and have a good time socially, with races optional.

In assembling this book, we have worked with members and officials of several clubs. For each region we cover, we have included a brief introduction to the major clubs there. The list is not exhaustive. We have focused on clubs with a broad following and an open membership policy, and limited our coverage to those clubs willing to contribute their information to us. If you do not find the club that best works for you in our list, please look beyond that list.

The New York City Marathon

The premier running event in New York City is the New York City Marathon, run every November, attracting more than 100,000 applicants and over two million spectators. The marathon, the product of the New York Road Runners Club, was first run in 1970 as multiple loops of Central Park. In 1976, it was moved to an on-street venue touching on all five boroughs of New York City.

The current route starts at the Staten Island end of the Verrazano-Narrows Bridge, passes through Brooklyn and Queens, enters Manhattan via the Queensboro Bridge, circumnavigates the Upper East Side with a short diversion into the Bronx, and finishes in Central Park (see map following).

If you are interested in participating, the main ways to gain an entry are to satisfy qualifying time criteria, win your entry in a lottery, or qualify by being a New York Road Runners member and finishing a specified number of qualifying races and volunteering in the *preceding* year. See the New York Road Runners website for full details.

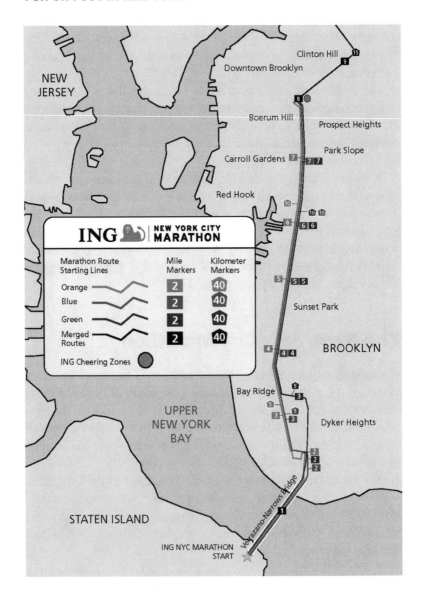

New York City Marathon Route, First Nine Miles

Copyright © New York Road Runners. Reprinted with permission.

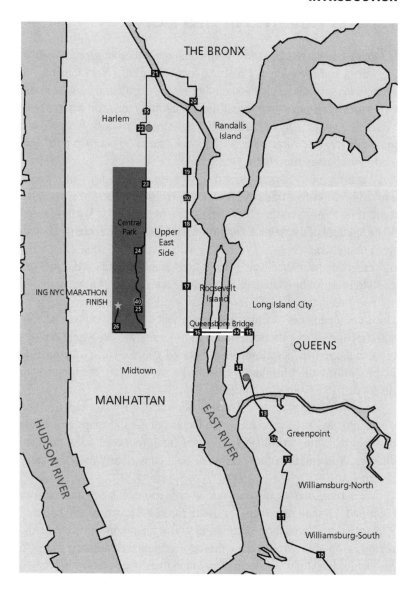

New York City Marathon Route, Last 17 Miles

Copyright © New York Road Runners. Reprinted with permission.

Places Covered in this Book

It would not be practical for us to catalog all nice outdoor routes in New York and New Jersey. We have focused on New York City and its immediate surrounds, plus some other major population centers in the two states. We have sought out the routes that meet our criteria best. We omit centers without sufficiently high quality routes. We have not generally targeted rural areas, so this book makes no claim to be a New York/New Jersey rural hiking guide.

We love New York City and have spent many days and weeks exploring its on-foot trails over the past 10 or more years. We have also toured New York State and New Jersey cities extensively. We developed all the content of this book from our own on-foot experiences (with help from many local contacts). We only document those routes that meet our criteria reasonably well. A few routes that we felt were just too good to miss we have flagged as *Fun on Foot Classic Routes*.

Some readers will likely enjoy following the exact routes we suggest. However, that is not essential and we expect many of you will take up some of the ideas presented and design your own enjoyable outings around them. In describing our featured routes, we try to provide helpful information for those readers who want to vary the routes with diversions, extensions, or shortcuts.

You may not want to carry this book around while out on foot. Therefore, we have produced a collection of all the maps and made that available for download from www.funonfoot.com for a nominal charge. You can therefore print your own copy of any map and carry it with you.

We apologize if we missed your favorite route. Please email us your ideas and we shall note them for use in future revisions of this book.

Let us now conclude the lead-in and embark on our tour of the region, with the comfort/attractions/convenience/destination formula as our guiding light. We start in Manhattan, the region's epicenter, and work outward through the other New York City boroughs and the city's immediate surroundings, ending with some more remote centers in Upstate New York and New Jersey.

Our main message: Get out on foot, get fit, see the best of New York and New Jersey, and—most importantly—have fun!

2

Manhattan

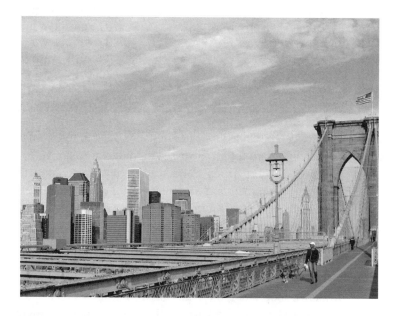

The borough of Manhattan, occupying a 24-square-mile island with a population over 1.6 million, represents New York City's heart and a big part of its soul.[1]

In Manhattan, on-foot is a common means of transport. Vehicles are very costly to operate and park, and not very efficient as a way to get around. The other option, the ad hoc combination of on-foot travel, public transit, and taxi, is frequently a better choice.

Manhattan has a simple geography, being a long, thin island, roughly two miles wide, sandwiched between the Hudson River and the East River. It is very easy to navigate, except possibly for the southern

---

1   Chapter head photo: The Financial District as viewed from the Brooklyn Bridge walkway.

(downtown) end, thanks to the grid system of numbered avenues and streets established in the visionary Commissioners' Plan of 1811.

We have put together some featured routes that we believe will enthuse any resident or visitor who likes on-foot action. In this chapter, we describe those routes that are entirely within Manhattan.

Route	Distance
MH1 Central Park	Various
MH2 Central-Morningside Parks Corridor	4.6 miles one way
MH3 Upper Hudson River and the Cloisters	4.5 miles one way
MH4 Mid-Upper Hudson River	3.9 miles one way
MH5 Lower Hudson River	4.9 miles one way
MH6 Lower East River	4.8 miles one way
MH7 Upper East River	4.2 miles one way
MH8 Harlem Parks Corridor	4.0 miles one way
MH9 Roosevelt Island	3.5 miles loop

These routes can be linked together in many ways to form longer routes. A few suggestions for people based in Midtown are:

- Midtown to Fort Tryon Park heading upstream along the Hudson River, returning via subway; 9.1 miles combining routes MH2 (Central-Morningside Parks Corridor) and MH3 (Upper Hudson River and the Cloisters);

- Midtown loop taking in Central Park and the Hudson River; 8.5 miles combining routes MH2 (Central-Morningside Parks Corridor) and MH4 (Mid-Upper Hudson River);

- Midtown loop along the Hudson River to Battery Park and returning along the East River; 9.7 miles combining routes MH5 (Lower Hudson River) and MH6 (Lower East River);

- Midtown loop taking in Central Park, the Hudson River to Battery Park, and the East River; 18.2 miles combining routes MH2 (Central-Morningside Parks Corridor), MH4 (Mid-Upper Hudson River), MH5 (Lower Hudson River), and MH6 (Lower East River).

Subsequent chapters include some routes extending from Manhattan into other New York City boroughs or adjacent New Jersey. They include routes over the Brooklyn Bridge, Manhattan Bridge, Queensboro Bridge, Triborough Bridge, and George Washington Bridge.

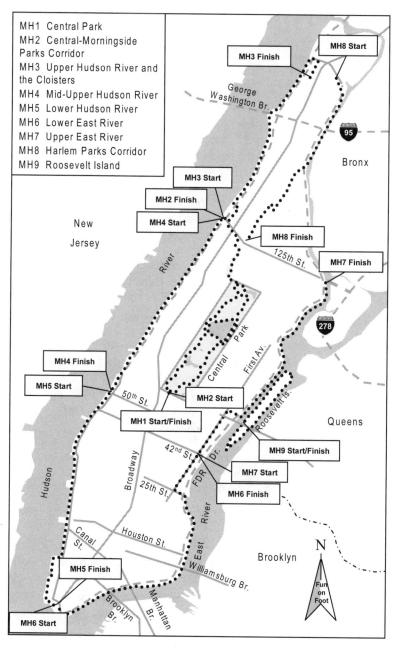

MH1 Central Park
MH2 Central-Morningside
Parks Corridor
MH3 Upper Hudson River and
the Cloisters
MH4 Mid-Upper Hudson River
MH5 Lower Hudson River
MH6 Lower East River
MH7 Upper East River
MH8 Harlem Parks Corridor
MH9 Roosevelt Island

Manhattan Routes

Central Park

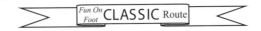

Distance	Various (Route MH1)
Comfort	Excellent underfoot conditions in the park, on a path or in a lane dedicated to pedestrians. Expect many on-foot exercisers, cyclists, and others around but there is plenty of room for all. On most park roads, there are no vehicles on weekends or off-peak most weekdays. The Park Drive loop is good for inline skating.
Attractions	Beautifully landscaped green space, varied terrain, varied vegetation, and several attractive lakes. A number of points of interest (see map).
Convenience	On-foot routes are convenient to all Midtown hotels, and addresses on the Upper West Side and Upper East Side. There are several subway stations handy, giving access to all major north-south subway lines, connecting to Lower Manhattan, Brooklyn, and the Bronx. Stations for east-west subway lines to Queens are also nearby. We describe our main featured route starting and finishing in Midtown at the park's south boundary.
Destination	Pick your favorite Midtown or Uptown destination. There are innumerable casual food or beverage destinations, for example, in the nearby theatre district or the Upper West Side.

While I do not have the statistics to prove it, I have no doubt this is the most popular on-foot exercise place in the world. It is standard fare for locals and fitness-conscious visitors alike. It is also of special significance to runners, being the finish point for the famous New York City Marathon. It is also the location of many races and fun runs, including the popular four-mile Midnight Run which starts when the clock strikes twelve on New Years Eve.

Central Park is a 2.5-mile by 0.5-mile tasteful nature preserve, bang in the middle of the densest population region of the country. It is easily

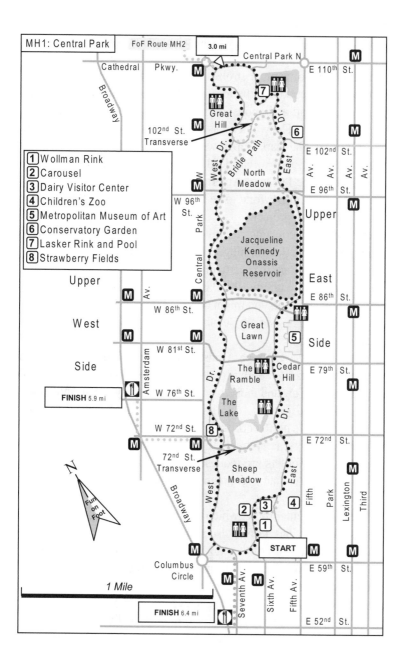

reached on-foot from any hotel or residence in Midtown, the Upper West Side, or the Upper East Side.

Interestingly, Central Park was not a part of the Commissioners' Plan of 1811 that established the master street plan for Manhattan. Rather, it was the result of another stroke of planning brilliance in 1853, when the city leaders endorsed the idea of a large, central public park. The city acquired land and sponsored a public competition to design the new Central Park. The winner was the "Greensward Plan" of Frederick Law Olmsted, the park superintendent, and local architect Calvert Vaux. Olmsted, born in Hartford Connecticut, subsequently became recognized as the father of American landscape architecture. Central Park was his first great work, to be followed later by several other major urban landscaping projects.

Central Park contains 58 miles of pedestrian paths, not all of which are suitable for running because of crowds of slow people in some parts. There are two particularly popular routes for runners—the reservoir jogging path and the Park Drive loop. The bridle path (see map) is another option you might consider. There are restrooms spread throughout the park, and ample other facilities such as food outlets and water fountains.

The Jacqueline Kennedy Onassis Reservoir occupies most of the width of the park from 86th Street to 96th Street. There is a 1.58-mile soft jogging path around the reservoir, which is very scenic and popular with runners and joggers. On this loop, you get beautiful views of Midtown from the north end. In May you are treated to an environment of flowering pink cherry trees. Bicycles, inline skates, and dogs are prohibited. On-footers are requested to go counterclockwise, and the majority adhere to that. You can access this path at many different points around it.

The other popular route, which we feature in more detail, is the 6.1-mile road circuit, Park Drive (also known as West Drive and East Drive on the respective sides of the park). This road is closed to vehicles on weekends year-round and in off-peak hours on weekdays except from Thanksgiving through New Year. When closed to vehicles, it is used by large numbers of on-foot exercisers, cyclists, inline skaters, and strolling pedestrians, but there is plenty of room for all. Even when it is open to vehicles, its side recreation path is fine for runners and walkers.

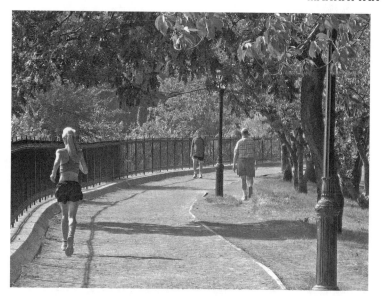

The Reservoir Jogging Path

The vehicular traffic (if any) and bicycle traffic travel counterclockwise around the loop. Most pedestrians go that way too, although there is an argument that they should go the opposite direction to other traffic. We shall assume counterclockwise for our featured route.

Our assumed start-point is at Central Park South, another name for 59th Street where it borders the park. There are park entrances at Sixth (Avenue of the Americas), Seventh, and Eighth Avenues. You can easily get here walking or running from any Midtown hotel, or by riding any of several subway lines (get off at any 57th Street or 59th Street station).

Follow the road or path north a short distance until you reach Park Drive and then turn right. There are many things you may want to see in Central Park, and we shall not mention all of them. One place you might want to swing by near the start of your route is the Dairy. It is down a path to the right off Park Drive, where you can see the 1908-vintage carousel on the left. The Dairy contains an information center where you can obtain a free detailed map of the park.

Continue following the road, which takes you past the Metropolitan Museum of Art. On the left you pass the Great Lawn, formerly the Lower Croton reservoir until it was filled in 1937.

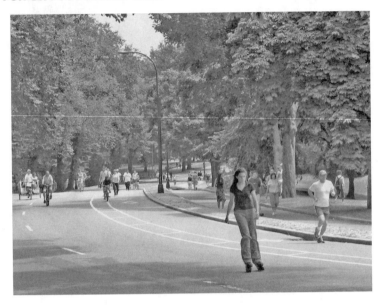

Typical Weekend Scene on Park Drive

You then come to the Jacqueline Kennedy Onassis Reservoir. After the reservoir, Park Drive takes you through the large North Meadow area, and you pass the Conservatory Garden to your right. In due course you arrive near the north edge of the park at 110th Street. Keep following Park Drive as it circles back southward near the western boundary of the park. Pass Great Hill (or Harlem Hill), an excellent place to work out if you want some grades.

Follow West Drive south to your exit point (or keep going and do another loop if you are in a 12-mile frame of mind).

We can suggest two nice exit points. The first is at W 72nd Street. This is near Strawberry Fields, the beautifully landscaped garden of international peace dedicated to the memory of John Lennon. You should walk through it if you have not been here before.

Nola and I happened to be running in Central Park the day after George Harrison's death and were somehow drawn to Strawberry Fields. It turned out we were far from alone—many of the Beatles' faithful made their way to the same place to pay their respects at a spontaneous, peaceful memorial for the loss of a second Beatle.

If you exit the park at W 72nd Street and are ready for lunch or a drink, you are close to an excellent West Side eating and drinking area. Head west two avenues to Amsterdam Avenue. There are several good establishments around here.

CENTRAL PARK LIGHT POLE NUMBERS

Most light poles on Park Drive have an identifying code that can be very useful in telling where you are. The code starts with E, W, or C, indicating if you are on the east side, west side, or center of the park. This is followed by two digits telling you the nearest cross street. For streets below 100th the two digits are the street number. For 100th to 110th Streets, the leading 1 is dropped. For example, a pole with a code starting W79 indicates you are near W 79th Street and one starting E09 indicates you are near E 109th Street. (Thanks to Russ Charlton for this pointer.)

The other obvious exit point is back at Central Park South where we started. From here, you have easy access to the many Midtown eating and drinking establishments between Times Square and Central Park. We are partial to Rosie O'Grady's on Seventh Avenue at 52nd Street. If you like Irish Pubs or old New York saloons (Rosie's claims to be both), go no further. The food at Rosie's is good and the atmosphere warm and friendly.

If you are into museums or art galleries, you might prefer to exit the park on the east side, around the Metropolitan Museum of Art, where such institutions are clustered. If you go on to Third Avenue, you can find several good eating and drinking places here and in the other avenues east of Third.

VARIATIONS

There are two other important paved paths that you can use to shorten the distance of the Park Drive loop. These are the link roads known as the 72nd Street Transverse and the 102nd Street Transverse, which join West Drive and East Drive and have marked, paved pedestrian lanes. The "Inner Loop" involves using both of these transverses in conjunction with East Drive and West Drive and has a total loop distance of four miles.

Central-Morningside Parks Corridor

Distance	4.6 miles one way (Route MH2)
Comfort	Good-to-excellent underfoot conditions with plenty of on-foot exercisers and cyclists around. Most of the route is on dedicated pedestrian/bicycle paths, but with a few blocks on street sidewalks. Not recommended overall for inline skating.
Attractions	Beautifully landscaped green space in Central Park and Morningside Park, providing an interesting connection from Midtown to the Hudson River trails.
Convenience	Start in Midtown at Central Park's south boundary, convenient to most Midtown hotels. There are several subway stations on the major north-south lines nearby, servicing Downtown Manhattan, Brooklyn, and the Bronx. Stations for east-west subway lines to Queens are also close. Finish on the Hudson River at W 125th Street, where you have a choice of heading north or south on the Hudson trails. (See subsequent route descriptions.) There is a subway station near the end of the route at W 125th Street and Broadway.
Destination	Consider this route a connector to a route with a more compelling destination, such as the Upper Hudson or Mid-Upper Hudson routes that are also described in this chapter.

While a loop of Central Park is an excellent outing, you can construct more comprehensive routes by combining a traversal of Central Park with use of the trails along the Hudson River. We here describe a particularly interesting connecting route from Central Park to the Hudson, to link with the start of either of our routes that follow the Hudson upstream and downstream, respectively. For example, by combining this route with route MH4 (Mid-Upper Hudson River), you obtain a very attractive 9.7-mile loop starting and ending in Midtown, convenient to the theater district and Times Square hotels.

We suggest starting off with a three-mile half-loop of Central Park, taking you to the northwest corner of the park. While you could start from anywhere in the park, we assume starting from Central Park South, as with our first route. The map shows a route following Park Drive in a

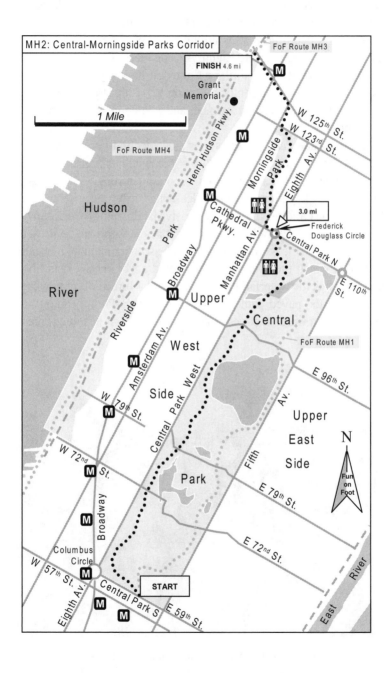

MH2: Central-Morningside Parks Corridor

FoF Route MH3

FINISH 4.6 mi

Grant Memorial

1 Mile

FoF Route MH4

Henry Hudson Pkwy.

W 125th St.

W 123rd St.

Morningside Park

Eighth Av.

Hudson

Cathedral Pkwy.

Manhattan Av.

3.0 mi

Frederick Douglass Circle

Central Park N

Park

Broadway

E 110th St.

River

Riverside

Upper

Central

FoF Route MH1

West

E 96th St.

Amsterdam Av.

Side

Central Park West

Av.

Upper

East

W 79th St.

Side

N

W 72nd St.

Fifth

Park

E 79th St.

Fun on Foot

Broadway

E 72nd St.

Columbus Circle

East River

W 57th St.

Eighth Av.

Central Park S

START

E 59th St.

clockwise direction, nearest the western boundary of the park, but you can choose a different route through Central Park if you wish.

Exiting Central Park at its northwest corner brings you to Frederick Douglass Circle, where Eighth Avenue meets W 110th Street, also known as Central Park North or Cathedral Parkway. Go around the circle and head one short block west on W 110th Street to Manhattan Avenue. Cross Manhattan Avenue, and you come to the entrance of Morningside Park.

Morningside Park (30 acres) has a decidedly different character to Central Park—much more of a locals' precinct than a place for everyone. In some respects that makes it more interesting. While it is not immaculately kept, it is generally pleasant. The big surprise in store in Morningside Park is some very impressive landscaping, which can rival Central Park's nicest hidden enclaves. It is less surprising to learn that this park is also the work of Olmsted. The scenery includes a beautiful waterfall, which the average tourist would never know exists. Note, however, that the waterfall is man-made and is turned off in winter.

Follow the paved path through Morningside Park, heading north and slightly towards the west. There is a restroom just after entering

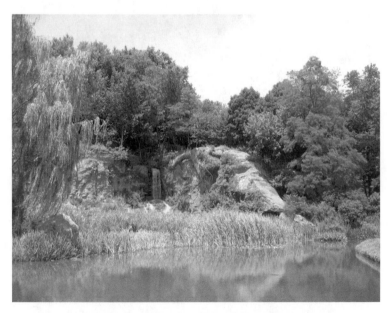

The Hidden Beauty of Morningside Park

the park. Exit the park at its northern boundary, W123rd Street, turn left, and head west a short distance to Amsterdam Avenue.

There are various ways from here to the Hudson River. All require traversing very ordinary streets for a few blocks.

We suggest going two short blocks up Amsterdam Avenue to W 125th Street and then follow that street to the left. (Alternatively, cut through the Morningside Gardens apartment complex to La Salle Street and Broadway, and then take Broadway northward to W 125th Street.) At the end of W 125th Street, take the underpass under the Henry Hudson Parkway to pick up the Hudson River Promenade.

VARIATION

Here is an alternative route to the river, starting from W 123rd Street and Amsterdam Avenue. It has the disadvantage of poorer underfoot terrain, including some hills, but it has some attractions of its own. Head westward up the hill on W 123rd Street. It will bring you to the tomb of Ulysses S. Grant, victorious Union commander in the Civil War and two-term President. Grant's tomb hides up on the bluffs above the river, in a granite and marble structure a little reminiscent of the Jefferson Memorial in Washington, DC. It remains the largest mausoleum in North America today. If you trek up here, to get back to our main route you will need to work your way north to W 125th Street to gain access to the Hudson River promenade. Alternatively, if you intend to follow the river downstream, head south and pick up the Riverside Park pedestrian trail along the top of the bluffs. You will later find linking paths down to the promenade.

Upper Hudson River and the Cloisters

Distance	4.5 miles one way (Route MH3)
Comfort	Good-to-excellent underfoot conditions with plenty of on-foot exercisers and cyclists around. The entire route is on dedicated pedestrian/bicycle paths. Suitable for inline skating in parts but not overall.
Attractions	The natural beauty and interesting sights of the Hudson River north of W 125th Street. The final part of the route is particularly beautiful, going through scenic Fort Tryon Park on the top of the escarpment. Optionally visit the historic Cloisters museum.
Convenience	Start at the west end of W 125th Street, where route MH2 (Central-Morningside Parks Corridor) ends. You can get here via the Broadway subway line (the 1 train). Finish at the 190th Street subway station (the A train). Trains from here take you back to Midtown (via Eighth Avenue), Downtown, or Brooklyn.
Destination	Visit the Cloisters museum or enjoy a food or beverage break at the New Leaf Café, before taking the subway home.

This route takes you upstream along the Hudson, north from W 125th Street, past the George Washington Bridge, to Dyckman Street. Here you can go up the escarpment and experience beautiful Fort Tryon Park and the Cloisters. Running conditions are excellent throughout.

Going north from W 125th Street, you may have to divert off the river onto the sidewalk of Riverside Drive to get up to W 135th Street. When we were last there, the West Harlem Piers Riverwalk was being constructed between W 125th and W 133rd Streets but that will hopefully be finished when you read this book.

At W 135th Street a paved multiuse trail starts up, but it is not on the riverbank. It starts under the highway and then drifts right of the highway. This trail section is a wide, excellent quality trail for runners, inline skaters, and cyclists, but it is not particularly attractive.

At W 145th Street, the situation changes. The path switches over to the riverbank and enters a pleasant recreational area, part of Riverside

Park. There is a playground here plus restrooms. Expect to encounter plenty of runners and cyclists. There are fewer access points back to the regular street grid here, but there is an access point at W 155th Street.

You then come to a sports field area and have a choice of path. The paved path goes right around the sports fields and an earth path follows the riverbank. The two paths meet after the fields. At W 165th Street there is pedestrian access to the street grid via an overpass, and there are restrooms.

After passing the tennis courts, go under the George Washington Bridge. Pass the little red lighthouse.

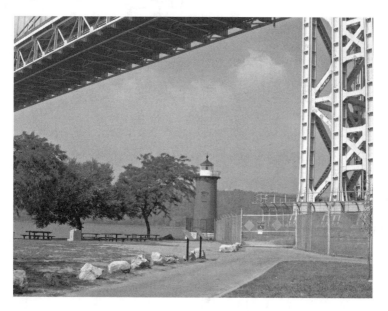

The Little Red Lighthouse Snuggling Under the GW Bridge

The path then becomes very peaceful for a while, winding through trees. It heads uphill and over the rail tracks, then under the southbound lanes of the Henry Hudson Parkway. It then starts following the northbound lanes of that road. It is not so pleasant here because of the vehicles zooming nearby, but the paved trail is still good quality.

There is an access ramp and overpass of the road at W 181st Street. Continue to the steps at Dyckman Street where this trail ends. Go down the steps and under the highway into Riverside Drive. If you need a

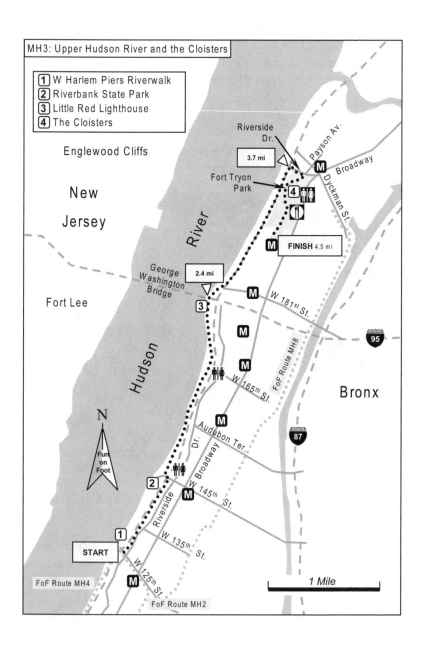

MH3: Upper Hudson River and the Cloisters

1 W Harlem Piers Riverwalk
2 Riverbank State Park
3 Little Red Lighthouse
4 The Cloisters

Englewood Cliffs

New

Jersey

Fort Lee

N

Fun
on
Foot

Riverside
Dr.

Payson Av.

Broadway

3.7 mi

Fort Tryon
Park

4

M

FINISH 4.5 mi

River

George
Washington
Bridge

2.4 mi

3

M W 181st St.

M

FoF Route MH8

M

W 165th St.

Bronx

Hudson

M

87

Audubon Ter.

M

Dr.

Broadway

2

M W 145th St.

Riverside

1

W 135th St.

START

W 125th St.

M

FoF Route MH4

1 Mile

FoF Route MH2

Dyckman St.

95

food or drink break go north a short block to Dyckman Street, where there are bars, restaurants, and a subway station.

VARIATIONS

From Dyckman Street you can easily connect to route MH8 (Harlem Parks Corridor), which takes you back to near the start of this route. This makes for an interesting loop route.

However, having got to this point, it is well worth visiting scenic Fort Tryon Park. At Riverside Drive and Payson Avenue there is a pedestrian entrance to this park.

Follow the trail uphill, generally bearing right. It is a little steep but excellent underfoot. You end up on top of the escarpment with excellent views over the Hudson River. As you approach the top of the path, you see the impressive classical building complex on the peak. This is the Cloisters, now housing a branch of the Metropolitan Museum of Art devoted to the art of medieval Europe. Divert to see it if so inclined or visit its public restrooms.

Continue straight ahead southward on the pedestrian trail along the edge of the bluff. You come to the New Leaf Café. If you want a food or beverage break, this is our recommended place for that. It has a beautiful environment, comfortable bar, and reasonably priced lunchtime meals.

After the New Leaf Café, continue a block south to the entrance to the 190th Street subway station. The A train from here takes you back to Midtown (via Eighth Avenue), Downtown, or on to Brooklyn.

Mid-Upper Hudson River

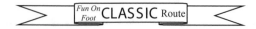

Distance	3.9 miles one way (Route MH4)
Comfort	Good-to-excellent underfoot conditions with plenty of on-foot exercisers and cyclists around. The entire route is on dedicated pedestrian/bicycle paths. OK for inline skating.
Attractions	The natural beauty and interesting sights of Riverside Park and the Hudson River.
Convenience	Start at the west end of W 125th Street, where route MH2 (Central-Morningside Parks Corridor) ends. You can get here via the Broadway subway line (the 1 train). Finish at the west end of W 50th Street, convenient to Times Square, Midtown hotels, and addresses on the Upper West Side. There are several subway stations nearby for the major north-south subway lines, connecting to Downtown Manhattan, Brooklyn, and the Bronx. Stations for subway lines to Queens are also close.
Destination	Many excellent pubs, restaurants, and other attractions around the theater district and Times Square.

This route mostly uses the trails of Riverside Park, a 323-acre park adjacent to the Hudson River from W 68th Street to W 155th Street. This park was developed initially in the last quarter of the nineteenth century and has been extended since. It includes sculptures and memorials exalting several of the city's heroes, plus many recreational facilities. Most importantly, it has excellent trails for on-foot exercise, with pleasant scenery throughout.

There are trails at two different levels. The first is the promenade (or esplanade), which follows the riverbank for almost the entire length of the park. You are alongside the water with views of New Jersey opposite. In addition, there is a trail, or sometimes multiple trails, inside the Henry Hudson Parkway. The latter trails largely use a corridor built over the buried Amtrak tracks going down to Penn Station. Below W 104th Street you can find various paths to switch between these trails. On your first time here we recommend using the promenade.

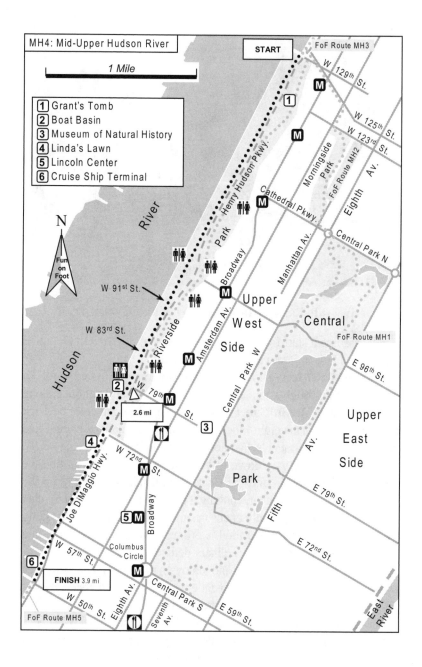

MH4: Mid-Upper Hudson River

1 Mile

START

FoF Route MH3

1 Grant's Tomb
2 Boat Basin
3 Museum of Natural History
4 Linda's Lawn
5 Lincoln Center
6 Cruise Ship Terminal

W 129th St.

M

1

W 125th St.

M

W 123rd St.

Morningside Park

FoF Route MH2

Eighth Av.

River

Cathedral Pkwy.

M

Henry Hudson Pkwy.

Park

N

Fun on Foot

Manhattan Av.

Central Park N

Broadway

Upper

West

Side

Central

W 91st St.

M

Riverside

W 83rd St.

Amsterdam Av.

FoF Route MH1

E 96th St.

Hudson

2

W 79th

M

St.

3

2.6 mi

Central Park W

Upper

East

Side

4

W 72nd

M

St.

Joe DiMaggio Hwy.

Av.

E 79th St.

Park

Broadway

Fifth

E 72nd St.

5 M

6

W 57th St.

Columbus Circle

M

FINISH 3.9 mi

Central Park S

E 59th St.

East River

W 50th St.

Eighth Av.

Seventh Av.

FoF Route MH5

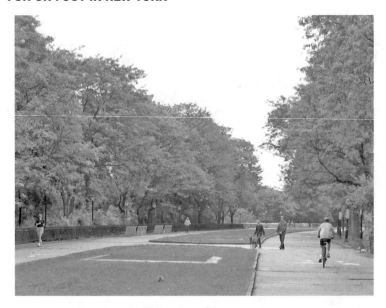

Riverside Park's Main Pedestrian and Cyclist Trail

We assume a start from the west end of W 125th Street. Go under the Henry Hudson Parkway to the promenade.

Proceed down to W 91st Street. Here you may be forced to follow the bike path through a tunnel under the highway, and continue along the upper trail to W 83rd Street, where you can take another tunnel back to the riverside. This eight-block gap in the promenade is being filled with a new trail segment, scheduled for completion in 2009.

Continue all the way down to W 79th Street. There you find the 79th Street Boat Basin and the Boat Basin Café. Depending on the time of year and the weather, you might find this a pleasant spot to relax over lunch. It generally only opens in summer and then not necessarily every day. If it is open, the food is ordinary but the atmosphere on a nice day compensates for any culinary deficiencies.

If you want to end here and enjoy a nice food and beverage establishment on the Upper West Side, you can exit Riverside Park at W 79th Street or W 75th Street and head two or three blocks east to Broadway or Amsterdam Avenue in the heart of the Upper West Side dining area. Here you will find many choices for eating, drinking, or both. After winding down from your on-foot exercise, you can easily walk back to your Midtown hotel or take a subway to other transit destinations.

Our route continues down the Hudson. At W 72nd Street a lovely area called Linda's Lawn starts. Linda was a long-time advocate for New York City park space. There are areas of ornamental grasses and boardwalks for pedestrians. The main bike trail goes under the highway and there is a separate pedestrian trail in many parts.

At W 58th Street the overhead highway comes down to ground and the paved bike trail starts to follow the roadway rather than being under it. At W 57th Street the pedestrian path separates from the bikes again and there is a little riverfront park.

From here on you are close to the busy roadway—you can cross it and get back to the Midtown street grid at many light-controlled intersections. At W 52nd Street, pedestrians rejoin the bike trail, near the cruise ship terminal.

We end this route at W 50th Street, where you can easily get to Times Square hotels, restaurants, and the subway. You are also close to the Intrepid Sea, Air, and Space Museum (see next route for more details).

Lower Hudson River

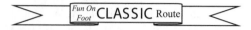

Distance	4.9 miles one way (Route MH5)
Comfort	Excellent underfoot conditions throughout on mostly dedicated pedestrian trails. No vehicle concerns. Expect plenty of other people about. OK for inline skating.
Attractions	Many cultural and recreational activities through-out, plus scenic views of the Hudson River and the Statue of Liberty. Specific attractions include the Intrepid Sea, Air, and Space Museum, Hudson River Park, the Irish Hunger Memorial, Museum of Jewish Heritage, the World Trade Center Sphere and eternal flame, and historic Castle Clinton.
Convenience	Start on the Hudson River, at or near W 50th Street, handy to the Theater District and Times Square hotels, the Jacob K. Javits Convention Center, and several subway lines. End at the south end of Manhattan, with convenient subway service to Midtown or Brooklyn, or ferries to Staten Island.
Destination	Battery Park and the Financial District, with many attractions and many excellent eating/drinking establishments for winding-down.

The Lower West Side of twenty-plus years ago, with its run-down docks and grimy industrial sites, is no more. Over the past decade this part of Manhattan's Hudson River bank has been transformed into a pleasant recreational area. Thanks are largely due to such initiatives as Hudson River Park, Battery Park City Parks Conservancy, and the Battery Conservancy.

When complete, Hudson River Park will be a 550-acre park stretching from W 59th Street down to the south end of Manhattan. At publication time, work is still in progress, but it is already a very enjoyable on-foot environment.

You can start out from anywhere in Midtown by heading west to the Hudson River bank. We nominally start at W 50th Street, a short walk from the Theater District and Times Square hotels. Proceed to Twelfth Avenue, cross that street, and pick up the paved trail heading south.

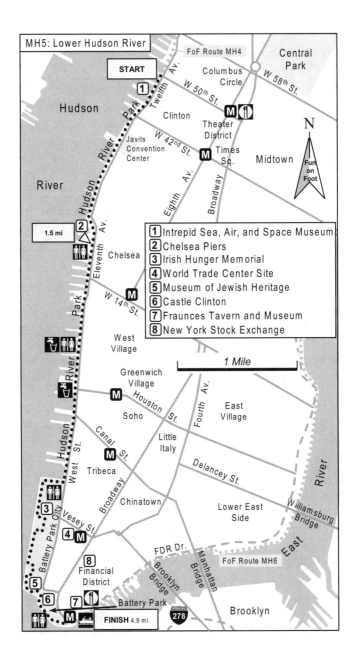

MH5: Lower Hudson River

START

Hudson

River

FoF Route MH4

Columbus
Circle

W 58th St.

Central
Park

W 50th St.

Clinton

Twelfth Av.

Theater
District

Times
Sq.

Midtown

N

Fun
on
Foot

W 42nd St.

Javits
Convention
Center

Eighth Av.

Broadway

1.5 mi

Eleventh Av.

Chelsea

Park

W 14th St.

West
Village

River

Greenwich
Village

Hudson

West St.

Canal St.

Houston St.

Soho

Little
Italy

Tribeca

Broadway

Chinatown

Vesey St.

Battery Park City

Fourth Av.

East
Village

Delancey St.

Lower East
Side

River

Williamsburg
Bridge

East

1. Intrepid Sea, Air, and Space Museum
2. Chelsea Piers
3. Irish Hunger Memorial
4. World Trade Center Site
5. Museum of Jewish Heritage
6. Castle Clinton
7. Fraunces Tavern and Museum
8. New York Stock Exchange

1 Mile

8

Financial
District

FDR Dr.

Manhattan Bridge

FoF Route MH6

5

6

7

Brooklyn
Bridge

Battery Park

278

FINISH 4.9 mi

Brooklyn

While the trail is sometimes shared with cyclists, progressively more pedestrian-dedicated parts are being built. The most northerly part is the least attractive, with considerable noisy traffic nearby. However, underfoot conditions are consistently good.

Proceed down to W 46th Street, where you find one of the most impressive sights of any city. Docked here is the *USS Intrepid* aircraft carrier, complete with a large collection of historic aircraft and other military relics on its deck. The *Intrepid* was in service from World War II through to 1974. Alongside it is the *USS Growler,* a strategic nuclear missile submarine (open to the public). This collection of sea craft, aircraft, and other memorabilia, known as the Intrepid Sea, Air, and Space Museum, is rounded out by a Concorde supersonic jet—not just any Concorde, but the aircraft that set the record for the fastest Atlantic crossing by any commercial aircraft (2 hours, 52 minutes, and 59 seconds).

VARIATION

If you want to visit the *Intrepid*, consider doing this route in reverse, starting out from Battery Park (the southern end of the 1-train line) and making this museum your destination. After exploring the museum, then simply head east to wind down at one of the many restaurants in the theater district, around Seventh or Eighth Avenue.

Continue south, past the heliport at W 30th Street, to Chelsea Piers around W 20th Street. The four piers here house an enormous recreation complex. There are public restrooms here.

A little further south, pass the nondescript remnants of Pier 54, where the *Carparthia* landed in 1912 with all 705 of the *Titanic*'s survivors. It is also where the *Lusitania* departed on its final tragic voyage three years later.[2]

As you approach the Greenwich Village part of the park, use the pedestrian-only trail along the riverfront, rather than the bike trail. On reaching Pier 45 near W 10th Street, conditions become excellent for the on-footer. Vehicular traffic is now well away, and the landscaping and views are outstanding. Pier 45 and the esplanade between it and Pier 46 were one of the first parts of Hudson River Park developed. The trail is pleasant and relaxing, with grass and shade areas, restrooms, and concessions.

---

2   See www.atlanticliners.com for more details.

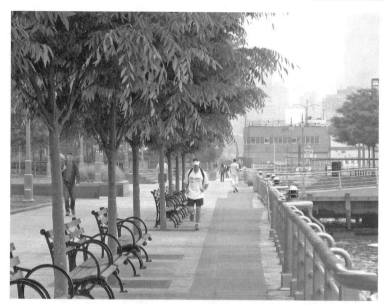

The Hudson River Park Trail

At Pier 40 near Houston Street, there is another pleasant recreation area, with various sporting facilities. Houston (pronounced *how-stun*, unlike that great city in the South) is the east-west street in Lower Manhattan that marks the end of the numbered street system. After Houston you get to see the Trapeze School of New York at work, flying through the air. Then, at Pier 25 near N Moore Street, you find the Children's Park and the Hudson River Sculpture Garden.

You then come to Battery Park City, a modern development on the lower Hudson comprising a tasteful combination of residences, businesses, and recreational spaces. Battery Park City is an excellent area for the on-footer, with the Statue of Liberty frequently in sight. First you take a sharp right to follow the river's edge. Continue to where you are forced to do a sharp left, around the edge of Governor Nelson A. Rockefeller Park with its large grassed area. At Vesey Street, you pass the Irish Hunger Memorial, remembering the 1845-49 Irish potato famine, when blight destroyed the Irish potato crop. Deprived of their staple food, over a million Irish died.

Continue past the North Cove Yacht Harbor, the esplanade where many community sports and other recreational activities are available, and then lantern-decorated South Cove. There are some restaurants and bars around here. Pass the Museum of Jewish Heritage and Robert F. Wagner, Jr. Park before leaving Battery Park City and entering historic Battery Park. For mileage purposes, our route ends at the lower end of Battery Park, at the South Ferry subway station.

In Battery Park there are various attractions including Pier A, the last remaining example of Victorian waterfront architecture in New York; Castle Clinton, an 1811 fort built to defend New York Harbor; and the World Trade Center Sphere and an eternal flame, memorializing the lives lost on 9/11. The Sphere was retrieved from the ruins of the World Trade Center. This is also where crowds line up to visit the Statue of Liberty.

You are close to the Financial District here. You can easily walk north to the World Trade Center site or northeast to the New York Stock Exchange, should you wish to visit them.

There are many places to wind down for some food and beverage around here. For a wide selection of food that you can consume in an outdoor seating area, there is the Amish Market at 17 Battery Place, near Battery Park. If you are more interested in a restaurant/pub, there are several excellent places in the financial district. Most notable is Fraunces Tavern and Museum, a short walk northeast of the park at 54 Pearl Street. Built in 1719, it is best known as the site where Washington bade farewell to the officers of the Continental Army in 1783. There is a casual bar area, as well as a more up-market restaurant. We can also recommend the cozy Ulysses Irish Pub at 95 Pearl Street or Pound and Pence at 55 Liberty Street.

To take a subway back to Midtown, there are various options. The simplest is the 1 train, which leaves from the South Ferry station at the lower end of Battery Park and roughly follows Broadway the length of Manhattan. The Staten Island ferry terminal is also here.

Lower East River

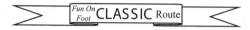

Distance	4.8 miles one way (Route MH6)
Comfort	Good-to-excellent underfoot conditions with plenty of on-foot exercisers and cyclists around. Most of the route is on dedicated pedestrian or pedestrian/ bicycle paths; the rest is on street sidewalks. Not recommended overall for inline skating.
Attractions	The fresh air of the East River and the scenic views across the river and of the famous bridges. Pass the Vietnam Veterans Memorial and pass through the Seaport Historical District.
Convenience	Start at the South Ferry subway station at the lower end of Battery Park. Get here via the Broadway subway (the 1 train) or Staten Island Ferry. End on the east side of Midtown, at the United Nations headquarters at E 42nd Street and First Avenue. This is close to Midtown hotels and Grand Central station, on the 4, 5, 6, 7, and S subway lines.
Destination	The United Nations headquarters is well worth visiting if no official activities are in progress at the time. Four blocks west on E 42nd Street is Grand Central Station, a transport hub and also a center for pubs and restaurants (especially E 43rd Street, west of Grand Central). Times Square is a short walk further west.

Our previous two routes followed the Hudson River. Manhattan's other river, the East River, also has a bicycle and pedestrian path for much of its length, except for a large annoying gap in Midtown. This route covers the lower part, which is the more appealing part. While this trail does not offer much in the way of big-city-escape, it does offer plenty of fresh air and impressive sights of massive skyscrapers and bridges.

We nominally start at the bottom tip of Manhattan, where our Lower Hudson River route ended, and finish at the United Nations headquarters at E 42nd Street. However you can equally well do this route the other way—both ends have ample pubs, restaurants, public transport choices, and tourist attractions nearby to help make for an interesting and enjoyable outing.

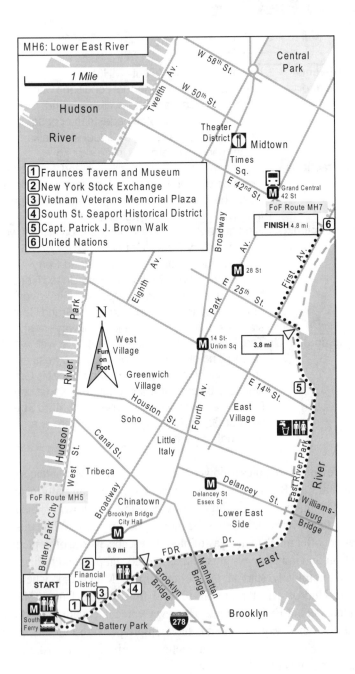

MH6: Lower East River

1 Mile

Hudson

River

[1] Fraunces Tavern and Museum
[2] New York Stock Exchange
[3] Vietnam Veterans Memorial Plaza
[4] South St. Seaport Historical District
[5] Capt. Patrick J. Brown Walk
[6] United Nations

W 58th St.
W 50th St.
Twelfth Av.
Central Park

Theater District
Midtown
Times Sq.
E 42nd St.
Grand Central 42 St
FoF Route MH7
FINISH 4.8 mi [6]
Broadway
Park Av.
First Av.
[M] 28 St
E 25th St.

N
Fun on Foot

West Village
Greenwich Village
Houston St.
Soho
Canal St.
Tribeca
Broadway
West St.
Canal St.
Little Italy
Chinatown
Brooklyn Bridge City Hall
[M]
0.9 mi
Fourth Av.
[M] 14 St-Union Sq   3.8 mi
E 14th St.
East Village
[5]
East River Park
River
Williams-burg Bridge

[M] Delancey St Essex St
Delancey St.
Lower East Side
FDR
Dr.
East

River Park
Hudson River Park
Battery Park City
FoF Route MH5

START
Financial District
[2]
[3]
[4]
[M] South Ferry
[1]
Battery Park
Brooklyn Bridge
Manhattan Bridge
278
Brooklyn

From the lower end of Battery Park, pick up the sidewalk of South Street heading east around the shore. There are restrooms at the Staten Island Ferry terminal. The first part of the trail is a good paved sidewalk. As you progress north, South Street expands in traffic volume, and becomes Franklin D. Roosevelt Drive. The sidewalk also expands, becoming a marked bike trail in many parts. Generally, there is plenty of room for bikes and athletic on-footers, despite some clusters of wandering tourists.

You come to the downtown heliport, on a pier extending into the East River. Across the street is the peaceful Vietnam Veterans Memorial, tucked between the Financial District high-rises.

Near the end of Wall Street, you pass the Wall Street Ferry Pier. Then you come to the start of the Seaport Historical District, spanning Piers 15 through 17. There are historic ships here and other tourist attractions. There are public restrooms at Pier 17.

You then pass under New York's famous National Historic Landmark, the Brooklyn Bridge. If you are a visitor, you absolutely must run or walk over the Brooklyn Bridge. However, it is not so easy

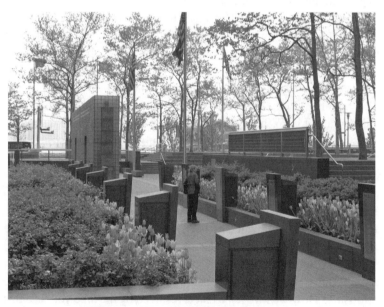

Vietnam Veterans Memorial Plaza

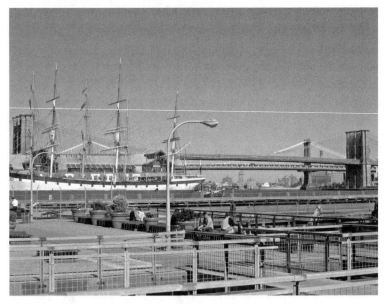

Views of Historic Ships and Bridges in the Seaport District

to get onto the bridge from the riverbank here. In the next chapter we feature a route covering that bridge, with full directions.

Continue up the river, under the Manhattan Bridge. You then enter East River Park, where the path takes you under the Williamsburg Bridge.

The paved bicycle and pedestrian trail up to E 18th Street is named the Captain Patrick J. Brown Walk. Patrick Brown, a renowned local military and FDNY hero, was among the New York firefighters that bravely sacrificed their lives in the September 11, 2001 destruction of the World Trade Center. As an on-foot exerciser himself, in accordance with his wishes, his ashes were scattered along a trail in Central Park where he loved to jog. The Captain Patrick J. Brown Walk is such a fitting memorial, passing in the shadow of the Stuyvesant Town apartment building in which he lived, and just close enough to the site of the building in which he died.

Proceed up to E 25th Street. When we were last there, the trail from E 18th Street to E 25th Street was under development and a little confusing. However, we hope that is resolved by the time you read this book.

The biggest remaining issue is that the East River trail ends at E 25th Street and does not restart until E 63rd Street. Therefore, you need to leave the river, move west to First Avenue, and follow that street's sidewalk for this part of the East Side. However, this is not really bad, since there are few cross streets and modest traffic volume. You are also usually in the company of other on-foot exercisers who face the same situation.

We end this route at E 42nd Street, at the United Nations headquarters. This is a convenient termination point, handy to Grand Central and to Times Square hotels. Our next route continues north up the East River from here.

If you finish your outing here and are interested in a food or beverage stop, go west on E 42nd Street to Vanderbilt Avenue, immediately after Grand Central. Then go north one block to E 43rd Street where you can find a selection of good pub/restaurants.

Upper East River

Distance	4.2 miles one way (Route MH7)
Comfort	Good-to-excellent underfoot conditions with plenty of on-foot exercisers and cyclists around. Most of the route is on dedicated pedestrian or pedestrian/bicycle paths; the rest is on street sidewalks. A major detraction of this route is the proximity to Franklin D. Roosevelt Drive and the resultant traffic noise. Mostly OK for inline skating.
Attractions	The fresh air of the East River and the scenic views.
Convenience	Start on the east side of Midtown, at the United Nations headquarters at E 42nd Street and First Avenue. This is close to Midtown hotels and Grand Central station on the 4, 5, 6, 7, and S subway lines. End at E 120th Street in East Harlem, where you can walk to Lexington Avenue to catch a 4, 5, or 6 subway train or run to the northeast corner of Central Park.
Destination	There is no compelling destination in East Harlem, which is primarily a residential area. However, the subway is convenient and can quickly take you to Upper East Side or Midtown restaurants, bars, or attractions.

This route lacks the appeal of our other Hudson and East River routes, but is excellent for someone living or staying on the Upper East Side.

We nominally start at the United Nations Headquarters where our previous route ended. There is a gap in the East River trail here, requiring you to use the sidewalk of First Avenue from E 42nd Street up to E 63rd Street. However, there are few cross-traffic streets here, so this is not a major concern.

At or a little before E 63rd Street, move east to York Avenue. At York and E 63rd Street there is a ramp to get to the riverside trail. Expect to find plenty of other runners and walkers on this trail, although the proximity of busy Franklin D. Roosevelt Drive detracts from its appeal.

At E 81st Street there is some relief from the highway intrusion, as the trail moves to a level above the roadway. This raised trail continues

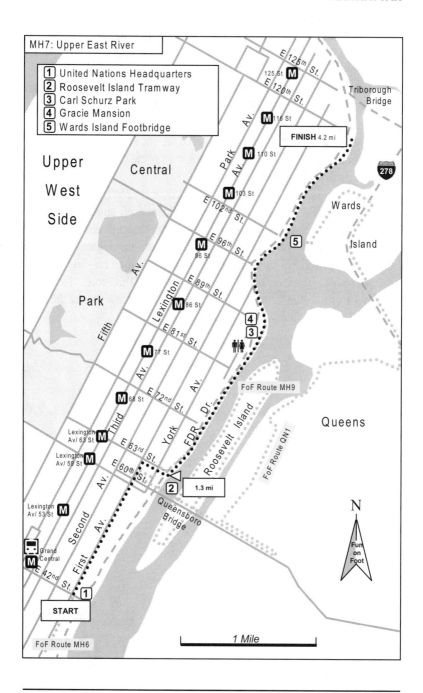

MH7: Upper East River

1. United Nations Headquarters
2. Roosevelt Island Tramway
3. Carl Schurz Park
4. Gracie Mansion
5. Wards Island Footbridge

Upper West Side

Central

Park

Fifth

Lexington

Av.

Third

Second

Av.

First

York

FDR Dr.

Park Av.

E 125th St.
125 St
E 120th St.
116 St
FINISH 4.2 mi
110 St
103 St
E 102nd St.
E 96th St.
96 St
E 89th St.
86 St
E 81st St.
77 St
E 72nd St.
68 St
Lexington Av/ 63 St
E 63rd St.
Lexington Av/ 59 St
E 60th St.
Lexington Av/ 53 St
Grand Central
E 42nd St.

Triborough Bridge

278

Wards Island

5

4
3

FoF Route MH9

Roosevelt Island

Queens

FoF Route QN1

2 1.3 mi

Queensboro Bridge

N

Fun on Foot

1 United Nations Headquarters

START

FoF Route MH6

1 Mile

on to skirt Carl Schurz Park—the environment is very pleasant here. Pass Gracie Mansion, the 1799-vintage official home of the Mayor of New York City. You can exit back to the main street grid at E 89th Street if necessary.

From this point onwards, the trail again follows the edge of Franklin D. Roosevelt Drive. The trail here is called Bobby Wagner Walk. There are accesses back to the street grid at E 96th Street, E 102nd Street, E 111th Street, and E 120th Street. At E 102nd Street you pass the Wards Island Footbridge, where you can connect to route QN1 (Queensboro-Triborough Bridges Loop).

The trail ends at the Triborough Bridge, near E 125th Street, but there is presently no access back to the street grid here. We suggest exiting at E 120th Street, where you can continue on-foot through East Harlem to Lexington Avenue. There are subway stations on Lexington Avenue at E 116th Street and E 125th Street. This is primarily a residential area. You can also continue on to Fifth Avenue and E 110th Street. Here you can enter Central Park at its northeast corner and follow one of the park trails back to Midtown.

Harlem Parks Corridor

Distance	4.0 miles one way (Route MH8)
Comfort	The first two miles are on a lightly used paved multiuse trail along the bank of the Harlem River. The remainder is on street sidewalks or park paths, but there are relatively few street crossings. The first two miles are good for inline skating but not the remainder.
Attractions	The fresh air and scenery of the Harlem River, the pleasant environment of Saint Nicholas Park, and the opportunity to touch the pulse of Harlem without becoming tied up in crowds or vehicle traffic.
Convenience	Start on Dyckman Street, near the top end of Manhattan, at the 1-train station (the A-train station is a little northwest of here). You can get here via route MH3 (Upper Hudson River and the Cloisters). Finish at W 125th Street and Morningside Avenue, where you can catch an A, B, C, or D train, or link up with route MH2 (Central-Morningside Parks Corridor) or MH3 (Upper Hudson River and the Cloisters). You can get from the finish point to the northwest corner of Central Park on foot via Morningside Park.
Destination	There is no compelling destination at the end of this route, but you can link up with our other routes or take a subway to your choice of Midtown or Downtown restaurants, bars, or attractions.

This route is not particularly obvious from a glance at the map but it is very good and has surprisingly few traffic encounters. It is particularly useful for someone seeking a loop route in the northern part of Manhattan—consider combining it with route MH3 (Upper Hudson River and the Cloisters).

Start anywhere on Dyckman Street and proceed east along that street, keeping to the left side. At the end, pick up the marked Greenway path along Harlem River Driveway. On the left you pass the entrance to Swindler Cove Park. Inside that park is the Riley-Levin Children's Garden, with public restrooms.

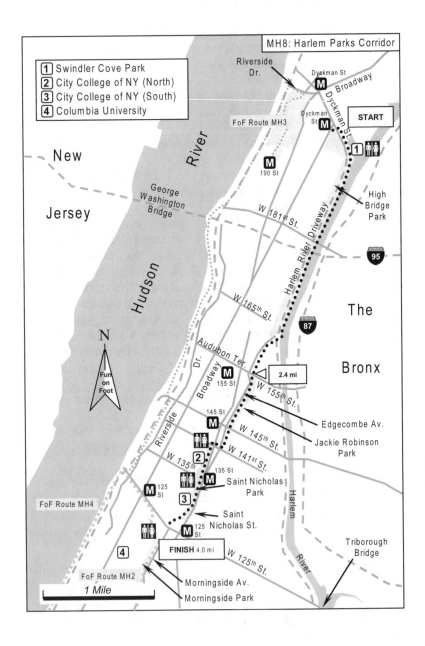

MH8: Harlem Parks Corridor

1 Swindler Cove Park
2 City College of NY (North)
3 City College of NY (South)
4 Columbia University

Riverside Dr.

Dyckman St

M Broadway

FoF Route MH3

Dyckman St. M

START

New

River

1

High Bridge Park

M 190 St

Jersey

George Washington Bridge

W 181st St.

Hudson

Harlem River Driveway

95

W 165th St.

The

87

N

Fun on Foot

Audubon Ter.

Broadway

Dr.

2.4 mi

Bronx

M 155 St

W 155th St.

Edgecombe Av.

Jackie Robinson Park

M 145 St

W 145th St.

Riverside

2

W 135th

W 141st St.

M 125 St

M 135 St

Saint Nicholas Park

3

FoF Route MH4

Saint Nicholas St.

M 125 St

Triborough Bridge

4

FINISH 4.0 mi

W 125th St.

Harlem River

FoF Route MH2

Morningside Av.

1 Mile

Morningside Park

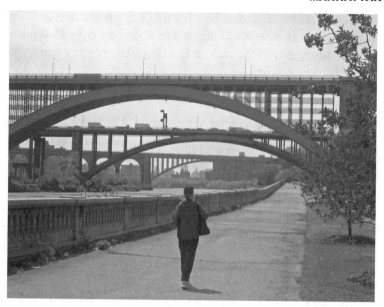

Harlem River Driveway Trail

VARIATION

As an alternative to using the paved trail along Harlem River Driveway, you can use paths up the bluff through High Bridge Park to get to W 155th Street. These trails are wooded, hilly, and sometimes confusing. We prefer the simple paved trail along the river but that is a matter of taste.

Follow the trail down the river. It is a very attractive trail in summer with serious attention given to landscaping. Pass under the three imposing overhead bridges which, among other things, carry Interstate-95 traffic between the Bronx and the George Washington Bridge to New Jersey.

The trail ends where the Driveway ramp to W 155th Street starts. Follow the signs up the ramp edge. Cross one traffic lane where required and continue uphill along the ramp to the traffic-signal intersection with W 155th Street. If desired, you can end your on-foot route here and catch a subway a block to your right on W 155th Street. However, we recommend continuing towards Midtown.

Cross W 155th Street and bear left into Edgecombe Avenue. This street follows an escarpment above Jackie Robinson Park. While it is not formally part of the park, it is an excellent running street with virtually no cross streets.

Cross W 145th Street at the traffic light. There is a subway station a block from here on the right.

Continue down Edgecombe Avenue to W 141st Street and go right one block to Saint Nicholas Avenue. Cross the intersection here to the entrance to pretty Saint Nicholas Park. There are restrooms here. Proceed through the park, noting the majestic buildings of City College of New York (North Campus) above the park to the right.

Climb the stairs and continue on the paved path south. At W 133rd Street there are more restrooms. At W 131st Street take the steps up the hill to the right to the edge of the City College of New York (South Campus). You come to a set of basketball courts—go left around them on the paved path.

The park ends at W 128th Street. Exit onto Saint Nicholas Terrace. Go right into W 127th Street and left on Morningside Avenue to W 125th Street. Our route ends here.

You have several options now. To the east on W 125th Street is a subway station to take you to Midtown or Downtown. To the south, at W 123rd Street, is the start of Morningside Park. There are restrooms here and you can follow route MH2 (Central-Morningside Parks Corridor) in reverse to get to the northwest corner of Central Park. Alternatively you can go west on W 125th Street to connect with trail MH3 (Upper Hudson River and the Cloisters) or MH4 (Mid-Upper Hudson River).

Roosevelt Island

Distance	3.5 miles loop (Route MH9)
Comfort	Good underfoot conditions with several on-foot exercisers around; bicycles are comparatively rare. The route is entirely on pedestrian paths or quiet street sidewalks. Not recommended for inline skating.
Attractions	The fresh air of the East River and scenic views across both sides of the river. A quiet environment without any of the road traffic intrusions characteristic of most of central New York City. Some historical points of interest.
Convenience	From Midtown or the Upper East Side, take the subway F train to Roosevelt Island Station, or ride the tramway from near E 60th Street and First Avenue. To start from the east end of Queens, use the Roosevelt Bridge from 38th Avenue.
Destination	There is no compelling destination on Roosevelt Island. However, the subway or tramway can quickly take you to Midtown restaurants, bars, or attractions.

This route is significant because it is convenient to Midtown and the Upper East Side but provides an excellent escape from the traffic and general bustle of those places.

Roosevelt Island (formerly Welfare Island) is part of the Borough of Manhattan but has a unique history. For much of the 19th and 20th centuries its main role was a place for charitable, correctional, and healthcare facilities. Since the 1970s it has evolved more into a residential park, but it still houses major hospitals and supporting institutions.

There are three ways to get to Roosevelt Island. The easiest is to take the F train to Roosevelt Island station. The most interesting is to take the aerial tramway from its terminus near E 60th Street and First Avenue. This uses technology more commonly seen at European ski resorts. The ride takes 4½ minutes, departures are frequent, and you get some excellent scenic views of Midtown and Queens. Furthermore, the tramway is part of the New York City transit system—passengers pay a nominal fare and can use their subway Metrocard.

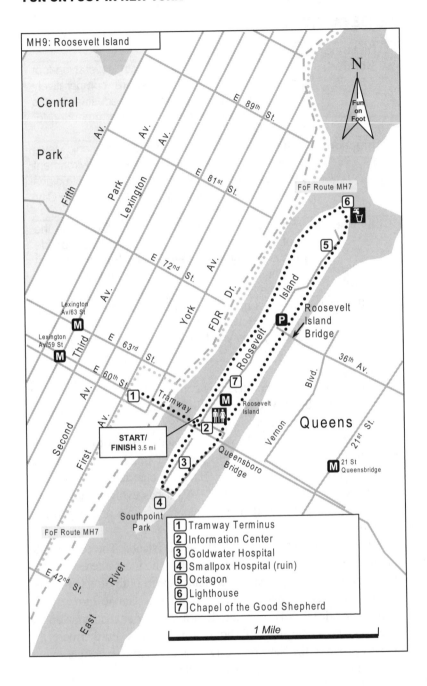

MH9: Roosevelt Island

1	Tramway Terminus
2	Information Center
3	Goldwater Hospital
4	Smallpox Hospital (ruin)
5	Octagon
6	Lighthouse
7	Chapel of the Good Shepherd

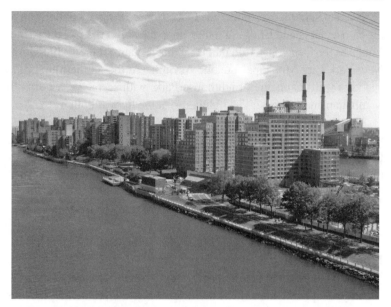

Roosevelt Island as Viewed from the Queensboro Bridge

The third way to get to the island is via the Roosevelt Island Bridge, from 38th Avenue in Queens. You cannot get to the island from the over-passing Queensboro Bridge, other than by negotiating some Queens streets to connect to the Roosevelt Island Bridge. We discuss that option in our Queens chapter.

There is a 3.5-mile loop around the island, connecting to all three of the access points. For description purposes we shall assume a counterclockwise loop starting from the tramway station. There are public restrooms and an information kiosk here.

Head south along the Manhattan side of the island, under the Queensboro Bridge. Pass the Goldwater Campus of the Coler Goldwater Hospital, on the former site of a massive penitentiary built here in 1832. You come to the entrance to Southpoint Park. When we were last here, the park was undeveloped and overgrown, although a project had been launched to redevelop it. There are scenic views from the park and some interesting ruins, including those of the 1854-vintage Smallpox Hospital. For our featured route, we chose to bypass the park for now, and simply follow the road along its edge to the Queens side of the island.

Head upstream, back under the Queensboro Bridge. Continue up to the Roosevelt Island Bridge and then up to the northern tip of the island. You pass the Octagon, a ruin that is all that remains of the 1839-vintage New York City Municipal Lunatic Asylum. At the northern tip of the island is well maintained Lighthouse Park, with scenic views of both Manhattan and Queens. The lighthouse at the tip was built in 1872.

Now swing back south down the Manhattan side of the island, with its views of the Upper East Side and Midtown. You pass, on your left, Roosevelt Island's Main Street area. Continue back to the subway or tramway station and take public transit to your next destination.

Running Clubs

Front Runners New York (www.frny.org)
This is a 500-strong running club for lesbians, gay men, and gay-friendly people of all athletic abilities. For 30 years the club has supported runners ranging from recreational walkers to competitive track athletes, road racers, and marathoners. Training is Tuesday and Thursday evenings and fun runs are Wednesday evenings and Saturday mornings.
Email: michaelabenjamin@gmail.com

Manhattan Track Club (www.manhattantrackclub.org)
The group usually meets in Central Park at 7:00 pm, on the Bridle Path near W 86th Street. The members run 8-10 miles most nights with one or two workouts per week. The club hosts the Bad Boy 5K/8K Cross-Country Race on the first Saturday in November, in Van Cortlandt Park, the Bronx. This club is well suited to serious athletes in training.
Email: info@manhattantrackclub.org

Mercury Masters (www.mercurymasters.org)
This is the only running team in New York exclusively for women aged 50 and over, seeking fitness, friendship, and fun. A few women have run ultras and many have run multiple marathons, but the club welcomes runners of all distances. More experienced members provide support and advice to less experienced members. The club meets weekly for a coached workout, and has group runs and parties throughout the year.
Email: alexabsmith@earthlink.net

Natural Living Running/Walking Club (www.naturalrunning.org)
This organization, associated with well known health and nutrition expert Gary Null, helps prepare athletes for the New York City Marathon in a fun, healthy, holistic way. The club focuses on good eating, good thought, latest training techniques, and training minus drugs. They meet weekly on Sundays in Central Park. They cater to runners, walkers, and race walkers.
Email: bigjonq@yahoo.com

New York Flyers (www.nyflyers.org)
This is a running club supporting the Upper East Side and Upper West Side, open to individuals of all athletic abilities and experience levels. It is also a social club. Demographics include all ages, male and female. The club hosts running, multi-sport, and social events including four seasonal parties. There are organized group runs every week, assorted fun theme group runs during the year, and long (marathon) training runs in September/October.
Email: info@nyflyers.org

New York Harriers (www.newyorkharriers.com)
This club, founded in 1988, has over 120 members who combine a passion for running with a zest for life. The team has roughly equal numbers of men and women, who range in age from early 20s to early 50s, some very fast, others not (all paces are welcome). The Harriers have an open membership policy, with a few tongue-in-cheek rules (see the website for details). There are at least two team workouts each week (speed work and long runs), and many social events year-round. Harriers combine a deep love of running with a friendly, accepting attitude toward others and a glint of fun in their eyes.
Email: nyharriers@yahoo.com

New York Road Runners (www.nyrr.org)
New York Road Runners, soon to celebrate its 50th anniversary, is dedicated to promoting the sport of distance running, enhancing health and fitness for all, and responding to community needs. Including the New York City Marathon, the club's road races and other fitness programs draw upwards of 300,000 runners annually, and together with a magazine and website support and promote professional and recreational running.
Email: Refer to website

Nike Central Park Track Club (www.centralparktc.org)
This is a competitive running club, open to all, covering road, track and cross-country. There are two coached workouts per week.
Email: webmaster@www.centralparktc.org

Park Racewalkers U.S.A. (www.parkracewalkers.us)
An organization dedicated to race-walking.
Email: Francicash@aol.com

The Reservoir Dogs (www.thereservoirdogs.com)
The club believes that with the right mix of training, rest and a great attitude, everyone can become a better and happier runner. Group runs and speed workouts are designed to accommodate a range of speeds and abilities, from sub-six-minute milers to 11-minute milers. Members' ages range from the low 20s to the mid 50s. Runners of all abilities are welcome at workouts. There are four group runs a week, and attendance varies from a handful to a crowd.
Email: membership@thereservoirdogs.com

The Roger Smith Running Team (www.rogersmith.com)
A team open to the employees, clients, friends, and hotel guests of the Roger Smith Hotel. The team runs in one New York Road Runners race a month.
Email: jfox@rogersmith.com

Warren Street Social and Athletic Club (www.warrenstreet.org)
Warren Street is a competitive racing-oriented social club that has been prominent in local races for the past 25 years. Membership and Tuesday night team training are free. The club meets in Central Park.
Email: Refer to website

West Side Runners Club (website in preparation)
A competitive running team with members from all five New York City boroughs, Westchester County, New Jersey, and Connecticut. The club has over 250 active runners who compete weekly in New York Road Runner races, plus other races in the tri-state area, the Boston Marathon, etc. Emphasis is on long distance running (half marathons, marathons). Membership includes some of New York's most talented runners including many Latinos and runners from Morocco, Europe, Kenya and Ethiopia, as well as Americans.
Email: dupontstaab@yahoo.com

3

Brooklyn

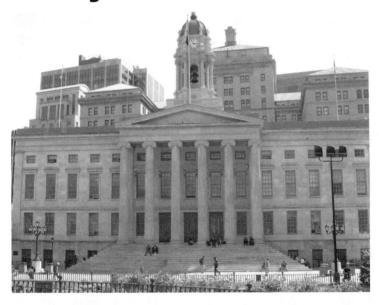

B rooklyn, home to almost 2.5 million people, has a history stretching back to 1646. In that year, the Village of Breuckelen was created by the Dutch West India Company and became the first municipality in what is now New York State (municipalities Albany and New York followed). In 1683, after the British had assumed power, Kings County was established here, along with eleven other counties forming the province of New York. Brooklyn was one town in Kings. All the pieces of Kings County were subsequently absorbed into the one City of Brooklyn. In 1898, that city merged with the City of New York, which before that time had only included Manhattan and the Bronx.[1]

---

1   Chapter head photo: Borough Hall.

From its origins until today, Brooklyn has been the chosen place for settling by a variety of cultural and ethnic groups. The resultant blend of diverse cultural sub-communities makes Brooklyn a place of tremendous character.

Brooklyn has some excellent running routes, thanks in part to its long coastline. Brooklyn is also convenient to reach from Manhattan, either on foot from Lower Manhattan or by subway from virtually any part of the island. Therefore, you do not have to be a Brooklyn dweller to consider running, jogging, or walking here.

We have selected nine Brooklyn routes, six of which are fully internal to Brooklyn. The other three involve connections between Manhattan and Brooklyn. The end points of all routes can be conveniently reached by subway.

Route	Distance
BR1 Brooklyn and Manhattan Bridges	3.9 miles one way
BR2 Brooklyn Bridge to Prospect Park	4.1 miles one way
BR3 Prospect Park	3.5 miles loop
BR4 Ocean Parkway to Coney Island	8.0 miles one way
BR5 Prospect Park to Bay Ridge	8.4 miles one way
BR6 Bay Ridge to Coney Island	5.5 miles one way
BR7 Canarsie to Sheepshead Bay	7.3 miles one way
BR8 Williamsburg Bridge	2.8 miles out/back
BR9 Marine Park	0.84 mile loop

These routes can be linked in various ways to each other and to the Manhattan routes to form longer routes. Some possibilities are:

- Starting in Midtown at E 42nd Street, reverse the final 3.9 miles of route MH6 (Lower East River) and tack on route BR1 (Brooklyn and Manhattan Bridges) to end in one of Manhattan's top eating and drinking areas; total distance 7.8 miles;

- Lower Manhattan to Coney Island via Prospect Park, returning via subway; 12.1 miles combining routes BR2 (Brooklyn Bridge to Prospect Park) and BR4 (Ocean Parkway to Coney Island);

- Lower Manhattan to Bay Ridge via Prospect Park, returning via subway; 12.5 miles combining routes BR2 (Brooklyn Bridge to Prospect Park) and BR5 (Prospect Park to Bay Ridge);

- A loop from Grand Army Plaza to Bay Ridge to Coney Island and back to Grand Army Plaza; 20.3 miles combining routes BR5 (Prospect Park to Bay Ridge), BR6 (Bay Ridge to Coney Island), and reversed BR4 (Ocean Parkway to Coney Island).

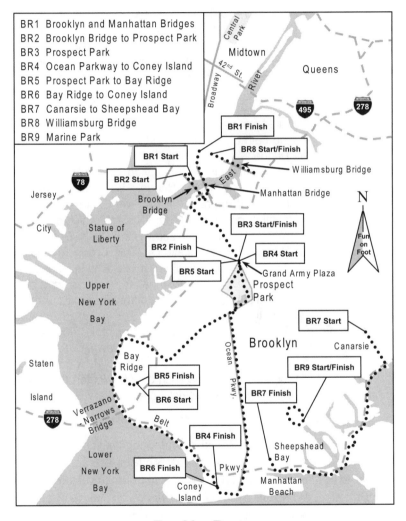

BR1 Brooklyn and Manhattan Bridges
BR2 Brooklyn Bridge to Prospect Park
BR3 Prospect Park
BR4 Ocean Parkway to Coney Island
BR5 Prospect Park to Bay Ridge
BR6 Bay Ridge to Coney Island
BR7 Canarsie to Sheepshead Bay
BR8 Williamsburg Bridge
BR9 Marine Park

Brooklyn Routes

Brooklyn and Manhattan Bridges

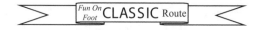

Distance	3.9 miles one way (Route BR1)
Comfort	Good-to-excellent underfoot conditions with many on-foot exercisers and cyclists around. Roughly half the route is on dedicated pedestrian or multiuse paths; the rest is on street sidewalks. There are some steps. Not recommended for inline skating.
Attractions	The fresh air of the East River and the unforgettable panoramic views of Manhattan while crossing both the Brooklyn Bridge and the Manhattan Bridge.
Convenience	Start in Downtown Manhattan, on the East River under the Brooklyn Bridge. You can get here on-foot using route MH6 (Lower East River). As another option start near City Hall, which can be reached via 4, 5, or 6 subway train to the Brooklyn Bridge City Hall station. (This option reduces the distance by about 0.4 mile.) End in Houston Street in Downtown Manhattan. You can walk or take a subway to Midtown or the Financial District from there.
Destination	The focal point for innumerable excellent restaurants and pubs in Chinatown, Little Italy, Soho, and Greenwich Village. Lower Manhattan tourist destinations such as Washington Square, the Financial District, and Battery Park are nearby.

If you have never crossed the Brooklyn Bridge on foot, you have missed out on one of life's great experiences. That is one of several compelling reasons to try this next route, even if you do not want to venture further into Brooklyn. While this route does not offer much in the way of big-city escape, it does offer impressive sights of massive skyscrapers and bridges and also the opportunity to cross two of those bridges and enjoy their spectacular views.

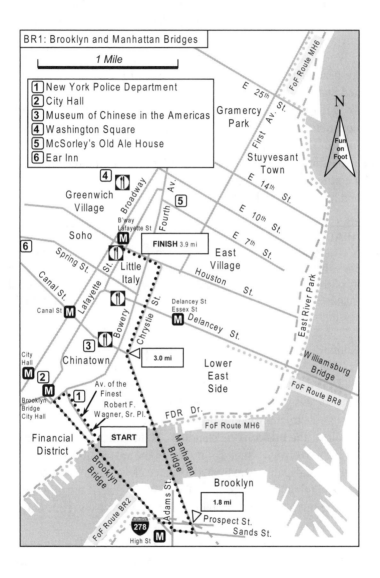

We nominally start under the Brooklyn Bridge on the East River trail (Route MH6), which allows you to easily link this route to a route either upstream (to/from Midtown) or downstream (to/from Battery Park).

Start at the first street upstream of the Brooklyn Bridge, Robert F. Wagner, Sr. Place. This street leads into the Avenue of the Finest. You quickly realize that you are now in the close vicinity of New York's police headquarters. This is probably one of the safest places in the United States.

To get up to the Brooklyn Bridge, there are steps near NYPD headquarters that take you up to a concourse with a big red metallic sculpture. Bear left past the sculpture and you encounter the start of the pedestrian path onto the Brooklyn Bridge. While this may all be a bit confusing, never fear since there are always many police officers around here who can direct you.

VARIATION

There is an alternative way up to the bridge, which involves more vehicle traffic but is less confusing. Use the street on the south side of the bridge, Dover Street, which leads into Frankfort Street. Continue up to Park Row and use pedestrian crossings to get to the pedestrian ramp onto the bridge.

Running (or walking) the Brooklyn Bridge is an unforgettable experience. This bridge, a National Historic Landmark, was opened in 1883. The intrigue surrounding the Brooklyn Bridge started with its enthusiastic designer, John A. Roebling, dying as a result of an accident during its construction and failing to ever see the result. For pedestrians and cyclists, the bridge is outstanding. Rather than using a sidewalk near a busy roadway, which is the case in the vast majority of bridges, pedestrians and cyclists are treated to a nice elevated pathway, amongst the cables high above the traffic. This not only keeps the traffic noise reasonable but also opens up panoramic views of New York City for the entire crossing.

You typically encounter many other pedestrians and some cyclists. On summer days, in good weather, tourists and tour groups can get in your way, so try to avoid those busy times if you are out for a serious training run. Be sure to pay attention to the signage and use the correct lane, to reduce the risk of being clipped by a cyclist.

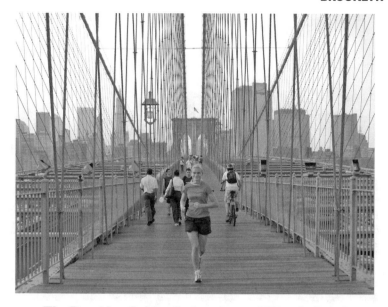

The Brooklyn Bridge Pedestrian and Bicycle Level

At the Brooklyn end of the bridge, the path splits. Take the left-hand, lower path. Go down the stairs to the intersection of Cadman Plaza E and Prospect Street. You are about to skirt the area known as DUMBO—from "Down Under the Manhattan Bridge Overpass." I kid you not—New York really has the most creative district names!

VARIATION

After crossing the Brooklyn Bridge, if you want to continue into Brooklyn rather than return directly to Manhattan via the Manhattan Bridge, see route BR2 (Brooklyn Bridge to Prospect Park). That route takes you to Brooklyn Heights, Downtown Brooklyn, and Prospect Park. You can take a subway back to Manhattan.

Follow Prospect Street westward, turn right at Adams Street, and then turn left into Sands Street. This takes you to the Manhattan Bridge. There are signs here to the bicycle and pedestrian walkways. The southern walkway is now dedicated to pedestrians only, the northern one being for cyclists only. You have excellent views of the Financial District buildings and the Brooklyn Bridge from the pedestrian walkway. (Once again pedestrians win out over cyclists.) The main problem with

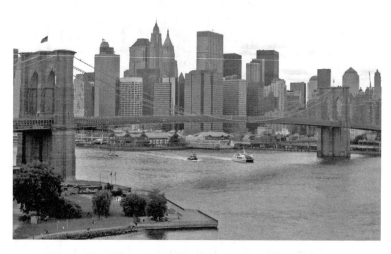

The View from the Manhattan Bridge

this bridge is the noise from both the vehicle traffic and the trains that use the bridge. Nevertheless, it is definitely a worthwhile experience.

The pedestrian walkway exits on Canal Street in the middle of Chinatown, so if you are ready for a Chinese meal your route has ended. However, there are also many other interesting restaurant areas within a short walk or jog of here. They include (moving progressively northward) Little Italy, Soho, and Greenwich Village. There are, in fact, way too many restaurants and bars around here for anyone to classify and compare them all.

VARIATION
To make this route a loop, from Canal Street take the Bowery south, back to the City Hall vicinity where the route started.

After much thought we decided to lead you to roughly the nucleus of this eating and drinking zone, which happens to be at our favorite Irish pub/restaurant in these parts, Puck Fair. This fine establishment is at the intersection of Houston and Lafayette Streets, in Soho. Houston, by the way, is pronounced "How-stun" and Soho means "south of Houston."

Washington Square, Greenwich Village, East Village, and Little Italy are all a hop and a skip from here.

To get to Puck Fair from the Manhattan Bridge, first go one block east to Chrystie Street, follow relatively sedate Chrystie Street north to Houston Street, and then turn left and head west a few blocks to Lafayette Street. Puck Fair is a top-class Irish Pub with excellent food, décor, and atmosphere. Its name reflects a pre-Celtic, goat-theme pagan festival still held annually in Killorglin, County Kerry.

There are also some very historic drinking establishments not far from here, if you like that sort of thing. A little northeast of Puck Fair, on 7th Street, is McSorley's Old Ale House, founded in 1854 and totally unchanged since, right down to the sawdust on the floor. The food is not the best by today's standards, but the place sure has character. Also, further west in Spring Street is the historic Ear Inn, built in 1817, and a renowned pub (or speakeasy) for sailors most of its life. The name "Ear" was adopted when the "Bar" neon sign partly burned out.

If you want to see the tourist sights of Lower Manhattan, such as Wall Street, Battery Park, or the World Trade Center site, all of these are an easy walking distance away.

There are many subway stations throughout this area. Alternatively, if Midtown is your destination and you have half an hour to spare, you can easily walk up there passing the Empire State Building on the way.

Brooklyn Bridge to Prospect Park

Distance	4.1 miles one way (Route BR2)
Comfort	Moderate running conditions. The first mile is on the Brooklyn Bridge pedestrian/bicycle path; the rest is on street sidewalks. Expect some other pedestrians around for the entire route, with a risk of crowds on the Brooklyn Bridge and in Downtown Brooklyn. Not recommended for inline skating overall.
Attractions	Cross the unforgettable Brooklyn Bridge, experience Brooklyn Heights Promenade with its stunning views of Lower Manhattan, pass through Downtown Brooklyn, and continue to Prospect Park, Brooklyn's answer to Central Park.
Convenience	Start in Downtown Manhattan near City Hall. You can get here by 4, 5, or 6 subway train to the Brooklyn Bridge City Hall station. End at Grand Army Plaza at the north end of Prospect Park. There are 2, 3, B, and Q train stations near here, servicing Manhattan and Brooklyn. This is also the place to embark on a loop of Prospect Park (see route BR3) or to proceed on-foot to Coney Island (route BR4) or Bay Ridge (route BR5).
Destination	Enjoy Prospect Park's pleasant environment, vehicle-free in off-peak hours in spring through fall. There are various eating and drinking establishments not far from Prospect Park.

For someone staying in Manhattan, this route serves as a connector to the on-foot gems of Brooklyn—the Brooklyn Bridge, Brooklyn Heights Promenade, Prospect Park, and routes beyond. We expect readers to use this route in many different ways to design enjoyable on-foot outings.

We nominally start at City Hall in Park Row, Lower Manhattan. This point is close to several subway stations and is a short walk from hotels in the Financial District.

Starting from City Hall, head east along Park Row and pick up the pedestrian ramp onto the Brooklyn Bridge. Ask a local if you have trouble finding it.

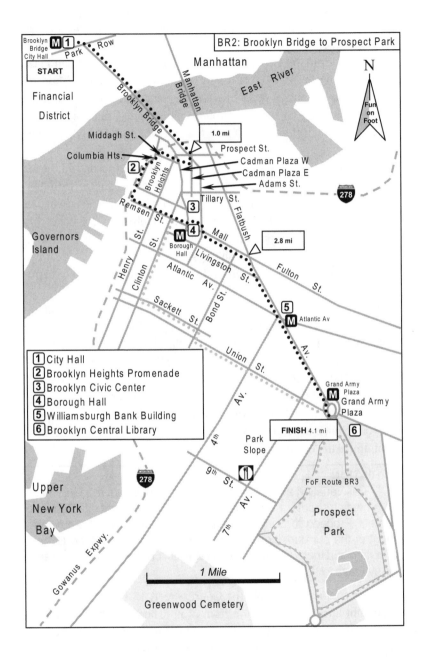

BR2: Brooklyn Bridge to Prospect Park

Brooklyn Bridge City Hall

START

Financial District

Manhattan

East River

Manhattan Bridge

Brooklyn Bridge

N

Fun on Foot

1.0 mi

Middagh St.

Columbia Hts.

Prospect St.

Cadman Plaza W

Cadman Plaza E

Adams St.

278

Brooklyn Heights

Tillary St.

Governors Island

Remsen St.

Henry St.

Clinton St.

Borough Hall

Mall

2.8 mi

Livingston St.

Flatbush

Fulton St.

Atlantic Av.

Sackett St.

Bond St.

Atlantic Av

Union St.

Av.

Grand Army Plaza

Grand Army Plaza

[1] City Hall
[2] Brooklyn Heights Promenade
[3] Brooklyn Civic Center
[4] Borough Hall
[5] Williamsburgh Bank Building
[6] Brooklyn Central Library

FINISH 4.1 mi

4th St.

Park Slope

9th St.

FoF Route BR3

7th Av.

Prospect Park

278

Upper New York Bay

Gowanus Expwy.

1 Mile

Greenwood Cemetery

Across the bridge, take the left ramp down where the promenade forks. Go down the stairs to the intersection of Cadman Plaza E and Prospect Street.

Go right from the staircase and then right again into Cadman Plaza Park. Follow the path, cross Cadman Plaza W, and enter Middagh Street. Follow it until it dead-ends and then continue on the pedestrian path past the Harry Chapin Playground. Go left into Columbia Heights and after about 100 yards you find the entrance to Brooklyn Heights Promenade.

Soon the scenic views of Lower Manhattan start to unfold on the right. At Orange Street a pedestrian trail starts—this is Brooklyn Heights Promenade, a beautiful and sometimes spectacular walk or run. There are outstanding views of Lower Manhattan. Expect plenty of people here, mostly promenaders but a number of runners as well. Bikes, inline skates, and off-leash dogs are prohibited.

At Pierrepont Street there are restrooms off to the left at the Pierrepont Playground.

The promenade ends at Remsen Street, a nice quiet street for running or walking. Remsen Street takes you directly to Cadman Plaza and the center of Downtown Brooklyn, where the quietness ends. Straight ahead is one of Brooklyn's most architecturally interesting buildings— Borough Hall, a Greek revival building built in 1849. It served as Brooklyn City Hall until fire damaged much of it in 1895.

There are many different ways to Prospect Park from Remsen Street, and your choice depends on your own tastes. Our featured route aims to minimize the distance.

VARIATION

This variation adds 0.4 mile but is more pleasant than the busy commercial streets. Take Clinton Street to the right off Remsen Street. Proceed to Sackett Street, turn left and enjoy the environment of the surrounding brownstone townhouses. At Bond Street, turn right and then left into Union Street. Union Street leads to Grand Army Plaza.

Cross Cadman Plaza W (or Court Street) to Borough Hall and go straight through the plaza in front of it. There is a subway station here. Bear right to the busy Adams Street intersection and the sign that heralds the start of Fulton Street Mall. Cross Adams Street to the mall. Follow either the mall or Livingston Street (one block south of the mall) to Flatbush Avenue. Both streets are shopping streets. The mall is restricted to pedestrians, buses, and delivery traffic. However, Livingston has much less pedestrian traffic, so might be the better choice if you are seriously trying to run through here. At Flatbush Avenue, turn right. The sidewalks of Flatbush are quite reasonable for running or walking, mostly passing by small commercial establishments. Head towards the Williamsburgh Bank Building, Brooklyn's tallest structure, and then follow Flatbush Avenue south to Grand Army Plaza.

Grand Army Plaza was originally decorated with just a simple fountain but is dominated today by the Soldiers and Sailors Memorial Arch. The arch, styled somewhat like the Arc de Triomphe in Paris, was designed by John H. Duncan, who also designed Grant's Tomb in Manhattan. The arch was completed in 1896. The Plaza now also contains a monument to John F. Kennedy and several other statues. The centerpiece Bailey Fountain, built in 1932 and recently restored, is a favorite backdrop in wedding portraits. A green market is held every Saturday, attracting many locals.

After passing through the plaza, you come to the north end of Prospect Park—see our next route description for details of this park.

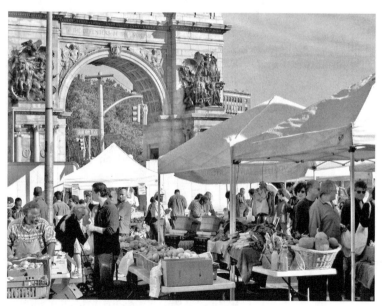

Grand Army Plaza Memorial Arch and Green Market

Prospect Park

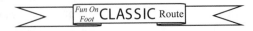

Distance	3.5 miles loop (Route BR3)
Comfort	Excellent underfoot conditions with plenty of on-foot exercisers and cyclists around. The entire route is on dedicated pedestrian or pedestrian/bicycle paths. Good for inline skating.
Attractions	A beautifully landscaped park with a variety of trails, ranging from woodland paths to roadways that are vehicle-free much of the time. Very popular with local on-foot exercisers.
Convenience	Start and finish at the park entrance off Grand Army Plaza, which has a 2 and 3 line subway station. Alternatively, start and/or finish at the Prospect Park subway station on the B and Q lines or the 15th Street or 7th Avenue station on the F line. If you are based in Manhattan, you can also get here on-foot via route BR2 (Brooklyn Bridge to Prospect Park). If you want to proceed on foot deeper into Brooklyn, you can go on to Coney Island (see route BR4) or Bay Ridge (see route BR5).
Destination	Enjoy Prospect Park's pleasant environment, vehicle-free in off-peak hours, spring through fall. There are various eating and drinking establishments not far from Prospect Park in Park Slope. If you head east on 9th Street from the Lafayette Monument, at 7th Avenue you will find a choice of food places and an F line subway station.

Immediately south of Grand Army Plaza is Prospect Park—Brooklyn's answer to Central Park. Olmsted and Vaux designed Prospect Park and Grand Army Plaza as their encore to building Central Park. The planning started in 1860. After the project was interrupted by the Civil War, the park was completed for opening in 1868.

At 526 acres, Prospect Park is roughly two-thirds the size of Central Park. Prospect Park fell into a bad state of disrepair in the middle part

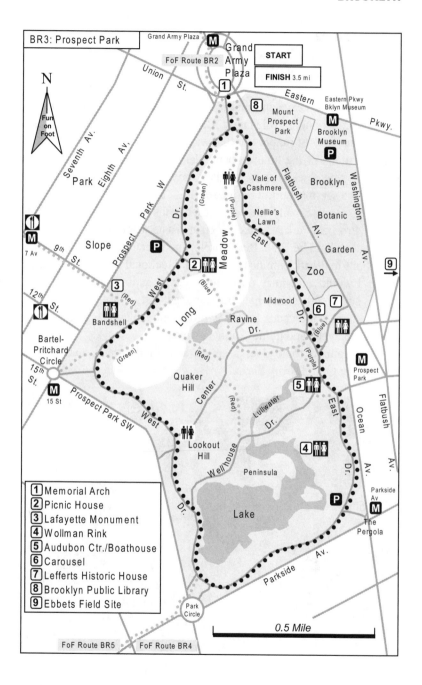

BR3: Prospect Park

START

FINISH 3.5 mi

1 Memorial Arch
2 Picnic House
3 Lafayette Monument
4 Wollman Rink
5 Audubon Ctr./Boathouse
6 Carousel
7 Lefferts Historic House
8 Brooklyn Public Library
9 Ebbets Field Site

0.5 Mile

of the twentieth century but, thanks to the efforts of the Prospect Park Alliance and the community, it has since evolved into a beautiful park which would make Olmsted and Vaux proud.

Similar to Central Park, Prospect Park has an internal roadway loop through it—3.35 miles around in this case. On the west side of the park it is called West Drive and on the east side East Drive. The loop has marked runner and bicycle lanes. Bicycles must go counterclockwise, and the majority of runners go that way too. The roadway is closed to vehicles much of the time; in particular, on all weekends and in non-peak hours on weekdays in February through November. The consequence is a set of beautiful on-foot exercise conditions.

There are also many other pedestrian paths through the park. Notably, the Prospect Park Alliance has created a network of four marked directional paths. The Blue, Red, Purple, and Green trails connect major attractions and park entrances. Colored directional arrows mark these trails. I would encourage on-footers to explore any trails found—the park is sufficiently small that you cannot get lost for long.

The park is the venue for many prominent athletic races, including running, bicycle, and inline skating events.

Our featured route does a single loop of the park, starting and finishing at Grand Army Plaza.

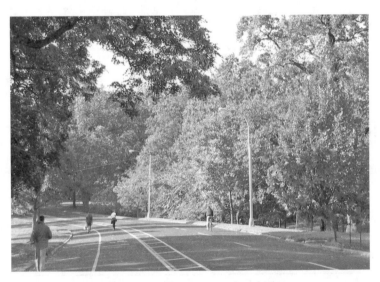

West Drive at a Vehicle-Free Time

Enter the park, passing the stately Brooklyn Central Library to the left. Then bear right on West Drive. One of the park's most important features is on your left—the Long Meadow, a 60-acre expanse of green grass that lays claim to being New York's largest open green space.

Pass the playground on the right and continue past the park maintenance and garage facility on the right. Then, before the band shell, you pass the crossing of the Red trail. The trail to the right here leads to the Lafayette Monument and the 9th Street park entrance. This trail is important to know, since 9th Street leads to some of the best food and beverage places around here, so you might want to head this way when you have finished your exercise. The next park entrance at 15th Street (Green trail to the right) also leads to good food and beverage places.

Continuing south you come to the scenic lake on the left. Pass the southernmost park entrance at Park Circle. This is where routes BR4 (Ocean Parkway to Coney Island) and BR5 (Prospect Park to Bay Ridge) start.

The road swings around towards the northeast here and becomes East Drive. Pass the Wollman Skating Rink on the edge of the lake and, after the Wellhouse Drive intersection, the Audubon Center at the Boathouse. The road heading off to the right here leads past the 1912-vintage carousel to the Lefferts Historic House, the zoo entrance, Flatbush Avenue, and the Brooklyn Botanic Garden.

VARIATION

If you exit the park east of the carousel and continue east beyond Washington Avenue to Montgomery Street and McKeever Place, you are where legendary Ebbets Field once stood. This was home to the Brooklyn Dodgers from 1913 to 1957, prior to their transplanting to California. Unfortunately, it is probably not worth the trip today, since just a plaque and apartment complexes fill the void resulting from the famous stadium's demolition in 1960.

If you continue north on East Drive, you will get back to the park entrance at Grand Army Plaza. Be prepared for a long uphill stretch as you approach the north end of the park.

VARIATION

Do more loops before exiting. Each loop is 3.35 miles.

There are many eating and drinking places around Prospect Park to drop into after a good exercise session. The best area is in Park Slope, off to the west of the park via the 9th Street or 15th Street entrance. F line stations are convenient to these places.

Here are some establishments that have been recommended by local runners:[2]

- *Café Steinhouse* at 14th Street and 7th Avenue;
- *Circles* at 15th Street and Prospect Park West;
- *Connecticut Muffin* at 15th Street and Prospect Park Southwest;
- *The Dram Shop Bar* in 9th Street between 5th and 6th Avenues (bar food);
- *Farrell's Bar & Grill* at 16th Street and Prospect Park Southwest;
- *Johnnie Mack's* at 12th Street and 8th Avenue (more a pub than a restaurant; serves pub food);
- *Le Petit Café* on Court Street near Nelson Street (specialty pancakes);
- *Mister Won Ton* at 7th Avenue and Berkeley Place;
- *Nono Kitchen* in 7th Avenue near 7th Street (Cajun/Creole, brunch);
- *Parco* in 7th Avenue near 15th Street (coffee, cake, croissants);
- *Smiling Pizza* at 9th Street and 7th Avenue (for an *amazing* slice of pizza);
- *Two Boots* on 2nd Street near 7th Avenue (Cajun, Italian, and an outstanding weekend brunch); and;
- *12th Street Bar & Grill* at 12th Street and 8th Avenue (more a restaurant than a pub).

---

2   Thanks are due to Alison Carrabba, Michael Balbos, Dave Mendelsohn, Rose Ann Serpico, the Brooklyn Road Runners Club, and the Prospect Park Track Club.

Ocean Parkway to Coney Island

Distance	8.0 miles one way (Route BR4)
Comfort	Good on-foot conditions. Expect other on-foot exercisers but no crowds. The route uses dedicated pedestrian or pedestrian/bicycle paths, plus sidewalks along a pleasant, spacious parkway. Not recommended for inline skating.
Attractions	Traverse Prospect Park, follow a wide runner-friendly parkway for 5.3 miles, experience suburban Brooklyn, and end at a famous amusement park and beach.
Convenience	Start at the Prospect Park entrance off Grand Army Plaza, which has a 2 and 3 line subway station. You can come on-foot from Lower Manhattan via route BR2 (Brooklyn Bridge to Prospect Park). End at Coney Island. There are D, F, N, and Q trains from the Stillwell Avenue station at Coney Island back to Downtown Brooklyn or Manhattan.
Destination	The country's most famous amusement park and fun area, Coney Island, including the historic Nathan's Famous hot dog joint. There are plenty of fast food joints but quality restaurants are scarce.

Do you yearn to visit Coney Island? Here is your big opportunity, seeing more of Brooklyn and gaining some fitness on the way.

This route starts from Grand Army Plaza. You can take the subway there or, if you want the 12.1-mile total distance, travel on-foot from Manhattan via route BR2 (Brooklyn Bridge to Prospect Park).

Starting from Grand Army Plaza, negotiate Prospect Park two miles to its southwest corner. See route BR3 (Prospect Park) for more details. Exit the park at Park Circle and follow the signs to Ocean Parkway.

Ocean Parkway extends for 5.3 miles from Park Circle to the seashore. It is a pleasant route for on-foot exercise. There are wide sidewalks on both edges plus additional pedestrian paths on traffic-separating nature strips for most of the way. There is traffic on the road, but being a parkway, no heavy truck traffic. You need to wait at traffic signals at many intersections but it is all very orderly.

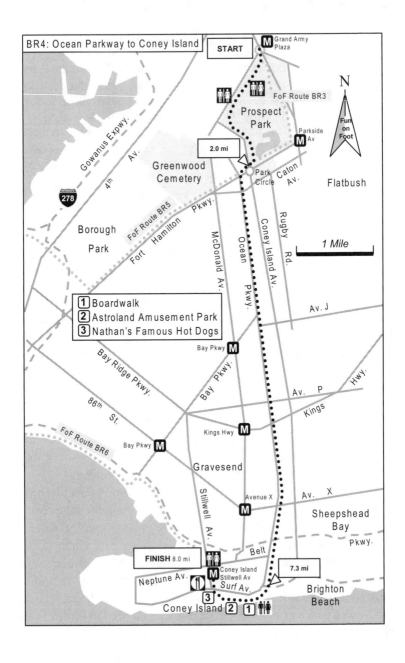

BR4: Ocean Parkway to Coney Island

START

Grand Army Plaza

M

N

Prospect Park

FoF Route BR3

Parkside Av

M

2.0 mi

Greenwood Cemetery

Park Circle

Caton Av.

Flatbush

Fun on Foot

Gowanus Expwy.

4th Av.

278

Borough Park

FoF Route BR5

Fort Hamilton Pkwy.

McDonald Av.

Ocean Pkwy.

Coney Island Av.

Rugby Rd.

1 Mile

Av. J

1 Boardwalk
2 Astroland Amusement Park
3 Nathan's Famous Hot Dogs

Bay Pkwy M

Bay Ridge Pkwy.

Bay Pkwy.

Av. P

Hwy.

Kings

86th St.

FoF Route BR6

Bay Pkwy M

Kings Hwy M

Gravesend

Stillwell Av.

Avenue X M

Av. X

Sheepshead Bay

Pkwy.

FINISH 8.0 mi

Neptune Av.

Coney Island Stillwell Av

M

Surf Av.

Belt

7.3 mi

Brighton Beach

Coney Island 3 2 1

Ocean Parkway takes you through a predominantly Jewish suburban neighborhood. While there are not a lot of exciting things to see, unpleasant surprises are very unlikely. This is an excellent route on a nice day.

VARIATION

Some local runners prefer the quieter side streets to Ocean Parkway, so you might want to try some other north-south streets as alternatives or mix it up. Rugby Road, a few blocks east of Ocean Parkway, was recommended by members of the Prospect Park Track Club.

There is not much in the way of facilities, either restrooms or refreshments on this stretch, so be prepared for that.

After passing under the elevated Belt Parkway, you come to the end of Ocean Parkway. We suggest either turning right on Surf Avenue, which takes you directly into the main Coney Island area, or continuing straight to the boardwalk and then turning right. The boardwalk, with its ocean views, can be very pleasant for running or walking. However, on summer days in particular, it can be very crowded, making running difficult. The annual Brooklyn half-marathon starts on the boardwalk.

The main sight you encounter is the Astroland Amusement Park, complete with its 1927-vintage Cyclone roller coaster. Coney Island was launched as an amusement resort in the early 1900s and reached its peak in the 1920s after the subway was built. Then, a million people a day would come here for fun. Today, it is nothing like that. The Depression, a 1944 fire at the Luna Park amusement park, and changing tastes and politics all took their toll. However, it is still fun for the young or young-at-heart, and rides such as the Cyclone make this place a living museum of fun activities.

Good eating and drinking establishments are not one of Coney Island's strengths. There is, of course, Nathan's Famous hot dog stand, still operating successfully since it opened in 1916. Nathan's is credited with originating the fast-food concept. It is at the intersection of Surf Avenue and Stillwell Avenue. There are also various greasy spoon joints throughout the area. There is a shortage of good mid-market eating and drinking establishments but you will not go hungry or thirsty. Regardless, when you have seen enough, you can catch the

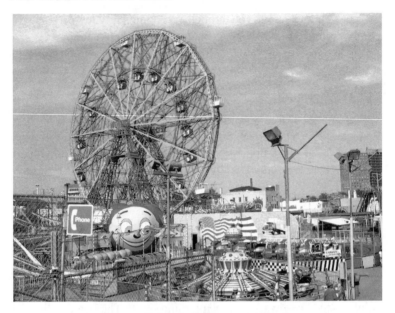

Coney Island Amusement Park

subway to Downtown Brooklyn or Manhattan, where good eating and drinking places abound.

The subway station is on Stillwell Avenue towards the western end of the amusement park, inland from Surf Avenue. There are public restrooms at the subway station.

If you like an eight-mile run, jog, or walk and also have nostalgia for old-style amusement parks, you will unquestionably find this route a winner!

Prospect Park to Bay Ridge

Distance	8.4 miles one way (Route BR5)
Comfort	Moderate-to-excellent running conditions. Roughly half the route is on dedicated pedestrian or pedestrian/bicycle paths; the rest is on street sidewalks. Expect some other pedestrians around for the entire route but crowds are unlikely to be a problem. Not recommended for inline skating.
Attractions	Experience the beauty of the Brooklyn shoreline, and touch the pulse of the diverse Brooklyn community. End in a lively Brooklyn neighborhood in the shadows of the Verrazano-Narrows Bridge.
Convenience	Start at the Prospect Park entrance off Grand Army Plaza, which has a 2 and 3 line subway station. You can come on-foot from Lower Manhattan via route BR2 (Brooklyn Bridge to Prospect Park). From the end-point in Bay Ridge, you can catch the R train to Downtown Brooklyn, Lower Manhattan, Midtown, or Queens.
Destination	Several excellent pubs and restaurants in the Bay Ridge region of Brooklyn.

As in our previous route, start from Grand Army Plaza and negotiate Prospect Park two miles to its south corner. See route BR3 (Prospect Park) for more details. At the park's south corner, an exit takes you to a large traffic circle, Park Circle. Follow the signs to Fort Hamilton Parkway, and take the right-hand sidewalk of that street.

You now face 2.5 miles along this sidewalk. The good news is that, since the street is a parkway, heavy trucks are prohibited. Furthermore, the sidewalk is wide and not crowded. The bad news is that the car traffic can be quite heavy. The enjoyment in this part of the route lies more in experiencing the variety of traditional life in Brooklyn than in any sort of scenic beauty.

After a few blocks, you reach the Greenwood Cemetery. Follow its southern edge to 37th Street. On-foot conditions in this part are very good, with no cross-street traffic.

The remaining 1.5 miles along Fort Hamilton Parkway, while not beautiful, illustrate Brooklyn's makeup very well. You traverse at least four distinct cultural sub-zones—eclectic, traditional Jewish, Chinese, and Middle Eastern. This is what characterizes Brooklyn!

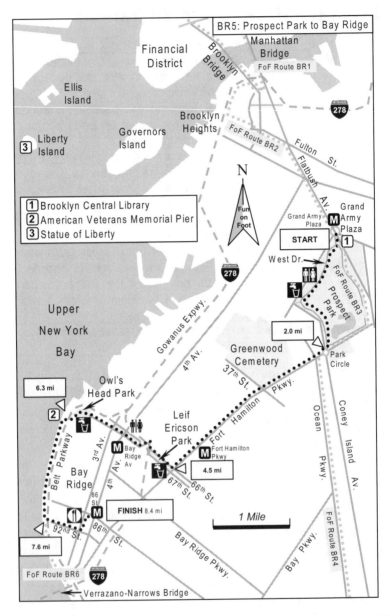

BR5: Prospect Park to Bay Ridge

Financial District

Manhattan Bridge
FoF Route BR1

Ellis Island

Brooklyn Heights

FoF Route BR2

Fulton St.

Governors Island

Liberty Island

3

1 Brooklyn Central Library
2 American Veterans Memorial Pier
3 Statue of Liberty

N
Fun on Foot

Flatbush Av.

Grand Army Plaza

Grand Army Plaza
1

START

West Dr.

FoF Route BR3

Prospect Park

278

Upper New York Bay

2.0 mi

Greenwood Cemetery

Park Circle

Gowanus Expwy.

4th Av.

37th St.

Fort Hamilton Pkwy.

Ocean Pkwy.

Coney Island Av.

6.3 mi

Owl's Head Park

2

Leif Ericson Park

Bay Ridge Av

Fort Hamilton Pkwy

4.5 mi

Belt Parkway

3rd Av.

4th Av.

67th St.

66th St.

Bay Ridge

86 St.

FINISH 8.4 mi

1 Mile

7.6 mi

92nd St.

86th St.

Bay Ridge Pkwy.

Bay Pkwy.

FoF Route BR4

FoF Route BR6

278

Verrazano-Narrows Bridge

The natural beauty re-emerges at 66th Street. Turn right into Leif Ericson Park, which occupies the land between 66th and 67th Streets most of the way to the shoreline.

Leif Ericson Park reflects yet another of Brooklyn's sub-cultures—the sizable Scandinavian-American community that settled in Brooklyn from 1825 through the rest of that century. This park is dedicated to the Norse voyager who landed in northeastern North America nearly 500 years before Christopher Columbus.

The park is decorated according to Norse themes. You might appreciate the water fountain at the entrance and restrooms further along at 5th Avenue. On-foot conditions are very pleasant, with plenty of shade and greenery.

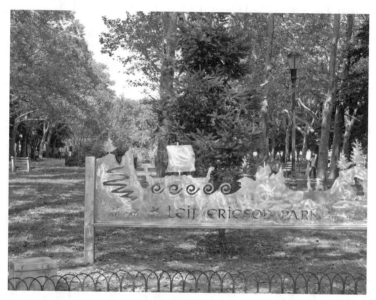

Leif Ericson Park Entrance

At 7th Avenue, there is a somewhat complex dogleg diversion that takes you over Interstate 278. There are pedestrian lights so no need to compete with road traffic. On the other side of the highway, pick up 67th Street and the continuation of Leif Ericson Park. Follow Leif Ericson Park to its end at 3rd Avenue. Continue following 67th Street two short blocks to Owl's Head Park.

There is a water fountain at the 67th Street entrance to this park. Negotiate this lovely park however you want—we found bearing left was easiest. You end up on the waterfront, with a view of Staten Island across the bay and, to the far right, the skyline of Manhattan and the Statue of Liberty.

Work your way to the southeast corner of the park at 68th Street. Here you find the start of a paved bike path. Follow that to 69th Street, and then turn right under the Belt Parkway to the American Veterans Memorial Pier.

Now you come to a wide, pleasant system of pedestrian and bicycle paths following the waterfront southward toward the Verrazano-Narrows Bridge. This bridge is of particular significance to the running community since it is the start point of the New York City Marathon.

At 1.3 miles after the Memorial Pier, take the pedestrian bridge over the Belt Parkway to 92nd Street. Follow 92nd Street to 3rd Avenue, one of Bay Ridge's two main streets. (4th Avenue is the other.) If you are ready for a break, there are some good food and beverage establishments here, with the Verrazano-Narrows Bridge tower always in sight.

VARIATION

If you want to continue on to Coney Island, rather than finish in Bay Ridge, do not take the pedestrian bridge but continue on the waterfront path. You are joining route BR6 (Bay Ridge to Coney Island). Linking these two routes this way gives a total distance of 12.3 miles from Grand Army Plaza to Coney Island.

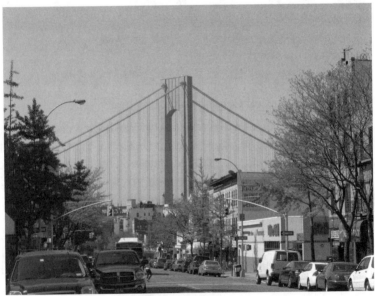

3rd Avenue, Bay Ridge

We like Henry Grattan's at 3rd Avenue and 88th Street—an Irish Pub with medieval-style decoration and very good food. However, there are many other places to eat and drink around here—we have no doubt you will quickly find something to your liking. Note you will be among locals here—not tourists. Bay Ridge is an excellent place to feel the pulse of Brooklyn in the very pleasant atmosphere of mid-market eating and drinking establishments.

To catch a subway home, go west to 4th Avenue at 86th Street or 95th Street. The trains from here will whiz you back to Downtown Brooklyn or Manhattan.

Bay Ridge to Coney Island

Distance	5.5 miles one way (Route BR6)
Comfort	Moderate-to-excellent running conditions. Roughly 3 miles are on dedicated pedestrian or pedestrian/bicycle paths; the remainder on street sidewalks. Expect some other pedestrians around for the entire route but no crowds. Not recommended for inline skating owing to rough surfaces.
Attractions	Experience the fresh air and beauty of the Brooklyn shoreline.
Convenience	Start in Bay Ridge, which you can get to by R train from Downtown Brooklyn, Lower Manhattan, Midtown, or Queens. End at Coney Island. There are D, F, N, and Q trains from the Stillwell Avenue station in Coney Island back to Downtown Brooklyn or Manhattan.
Destination	The country's most famous amusement park and fun area, Coney Island, including the historic Nathan's Famous hot dog joint. There are many fast food joints but quality restaurants are scarce.

Start at the 86th Street or 95th Street subway station in 4th Avenue. Navigate to 3rd Avenue and 92nd Street, and follow the latter street down to Shore Road, where there is a bridge over the Belt Parkway to the shore trails. Head left towards the Verrazano-Narrows Bridge.

Follow the shore trail under the spectacular bridge. There is a pedestrian sidewalk over the parkway at Bay 8th Street (Parkway Exit

4). On the other side is Dyker Beach Park, with sporting fields and a nice running trail around it.

At 18th Avenue there is a pedestrian bridge over the highway, leading to the Bath Beach neighborhood. There is a subway station about a half-mile up 18th Avenue.

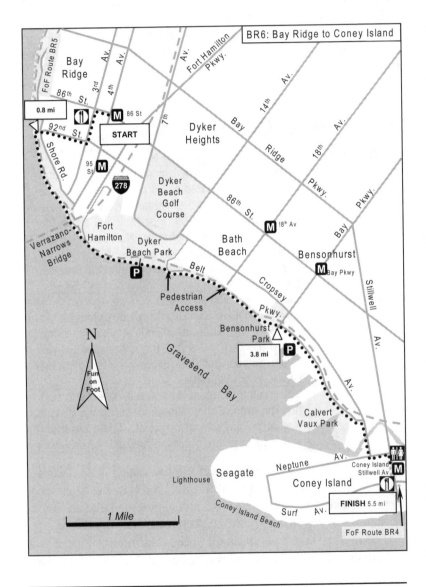

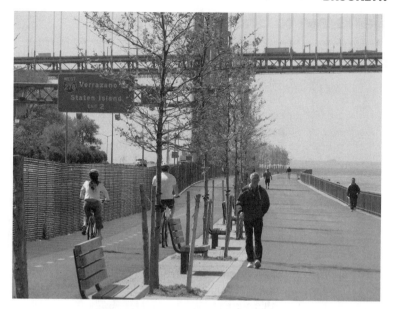

The Shore Trail Under the Bridge

Continue to the end of the multiuse trail in Bensonhurst Park, where Bay Parkway meets the shore. Here you need to pick up the street sidewalk that parallels the highway, with the shopping mall on your right. Pass the junior amusement park called Nellie Bly Park.

Continue past Calvert Vaux Park, which mainly comprises soccer fields, and continue to where the road splits. Take either split but bear left to connect with the sidewalk of Cropsey Avenue, where you turn right. Cross Coney Island Creek via the sidewalk. You now enter a very unexciting light industrial area, but the nation's most famous amusement park neighborhood is straight ahead.

At Neptune Avenue you can head left to the intersection with Stillwell Avenue and then right to the main Coney Island subway station at Mermaid Avenue. There are restrooms in the subway station. Alternatively, continue straight ahead to Coney Island Beach, the boardwalk, and the amusement park.

Good eating and drinking establishments are not one of Coney Island's strengths. There is, of course, Nathan's Famous hot dog stand, still operating successfully since it opened in 1916. It is at the intersection of Surf Avenue and Stillwell Avenue.

Canarsie to Sheepshead Bay

Distance	7.3 miles one way (Route BR7)
Comfort	Moderate-to-excellent running conditions. 4.4 miles are on a good quality, paved pedestrian/ bicycle path. The sections at both ends are on street sidewalks. Expect cyclists and some other pedestrians for the entire route but crowds are unlikely to be a problem. There is substantial road traffic noise from the adjacent highway for much of the route, but the traffic rarely interrupts your on-foot workout. Recommended for runners in distance training but not for people seeking a pleasant stroll. Mostly good for inline skating, except for the sidewalks traversed at the two ends.
Attractions	Experience the fresh air of the Brooklyn shoreline, on a good quality trail with few interruptions from vehicle traffic.
Convenience	Start at the Canarsie subway station at the end of the L line from Midtown. End in Sheepshead Bay, where there is a station for B and Q trains back to Downtown Brooklyn and Manhattan.
Destination	Sheepshead Bay is a lively center with pubs and restaurants and convenient subway access back to the main centers. You can alternatively continue on-foot a short distance along the sidewalks to Brighton Beach or Coney Island.

Brooklyn contains an excellent quality paved multiuse trail, which generally follows the Belt Parkway east of Brighton Beach. It stretches from Sheepshead Bay to the Queens line close to JFK Airport. It is not a particularly interesting route but it does offer a long uninterrupted run on a good surface, ideal for a runner training for distance.

This trail is not generally easy to reach, especially at the Queens end, unless you drive and park. However, the non-driver can reach it quite easily from subway stations at Canarsie (at the end of the L line) and in Sheepshead Bay, on the B and Q lines. Because the latter end is a much more interesting place to end a run, we have mapped out a route starting from Canarsie and ending in Sheepshead Bay.

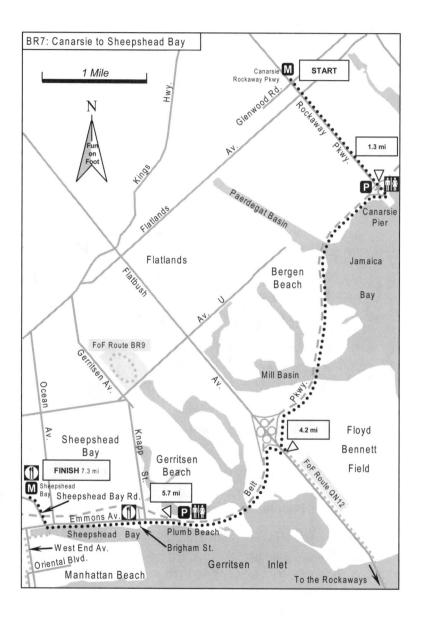

BR7: Canarsie to Sheepshead Bay

1 Mile

N

Fun
on
Foot

Canarsie
Rockaway Pkwy   START

1.3 mi

Glenwood Rd.

Rockaway Pkwy.

Hwy.

Av.

Kings

Flatlands

Paerdegat Basin

P

Canarsie
Pier

Jamaica

Bay

Flatlands

Flatbush

Flatlands

Bergen
Beach

Av. U

FoF Route BR9

Gerritsen Av.

Mill Basin

Pkwy.

4.2 mi

Floyd
Bennett
Field

Ocean
Av.

Sheepshead
Bay

FINISH 7.3 mi

Sheepshead
Bay   Sheepshead Bay Rd.

Knapp St.

Gerritsen
Beach

5.7 mi

Av.

Belt

FoF Route QN12

Emmons Av.

P

Sheepshead   Bay

Plumb Beach

West End Av.

Brigham St.

Oriental Blvd.

Manhattan Beach

Gerritsen   Inlet

To the Rockaways

Take the L train to Canarsie. Exit the station and bear left along Rockaway Parkway. This is a nondescript street with several fast food outlets and small grocery stores, should you need them.

After a little over a mile you reach the Belt Parkway. Go under it to enter the Canarsie Pier recreation area. There are restrooms here and many people on a nice day. There is ample parking if you need that. Pick up the paved trail heading south. In good weather, expect plenty of cyclists and a few serious runners.

The trail generally follows the Belt Parkway. The good news is that, being a parkway, there are no heavy trucks. However, it is a busy highway so always noisy.

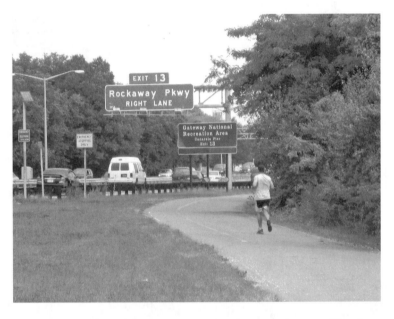

An Excellent Trail but the Busy Parkway is Always Nearby

The trail crosses bridges over two tidal inlets—the Paerdagat Basin and the Mill Basin—and narrows to a tight sidewalk on these bridges. However, the views are impressive and you experience plenty of fresh sea air at these points.

When you reach Flatbush Avenue, follow the trail around to the left. Flatbush Avenue southbound heads past the Floyd Bennett Field, with adjacent U.S. Navy and Coast Guard facilities, over the Marine

Parkway Bridge to Rockaway Park. While "the Rockaways" is a popular cycling destination, it is less attractive to Brooklyn runners because of the absence of an attractive loop route. However, you can do a combined subway and on-foot route between the Rockaways and Brooklyn—see Queens route QN12 (Rockaway Park to Brooklyn).

Shortly after the trail starts tracking Flatbush Avenue, there is a pedestrian/bike crossing with a traffic light. Cross and follow the trail to the right, back to the Belt Parkway. Continue to Plumb Beach. There are restrooms here and a very pleasant little beach. There is also parking.

Continue on and soon you will be delighted to see the highway veering away inland.

The trail ends at Brigham Street and you find yourself on the sidewalk of Emmons Avenue. This sidewalk is still quite good for running or jogging since there are no cross streets and few pedestrians. There are also some restaurants in Emmons Avenue, should you need food.

Continue to Ocean Avenue and pass the pedestrian bridge to the left across the inlet, heading to Manhattan Beach. One block after Ocean Avenue, Sheepshead Bay Road heads off at an angle to the right.

VARIATION

If you want to continue on to Coney Island, rather than finish in Sheepshead Bay, you need to travel roughly a mile along streets to get to the start of the Brighton Beach-Coney Island Boardwalk. Cross the pedestrian bridge over Sheepshead Bay inlet, turn right along the water's edge, turn left along West End Avenue, turn right at Oriental Avenue, turn left after a short block, and continue to the start of the boardwalk.

Sheepshead Bay Road leads you into the lively commercial center of Sheepshead Bay. There are various pubs, restaurants, and food joints here for a well earned break. From the Sheepshead Bay Station, catch the B or Q train back to Prospect Park, Downtown Brooklyn, or Manhattan.

Williamsburg Bridge

Distance	2.8 miles out and back (Route BR8)
Comfort	This bridge has excellent pedestrian and bicycle access, with a pedestrian-only walkway plus a shared pedestrian/bicycle path. Expect other pedestrians plus cyclists, but crowds are unlikely to be a problem since it is not a tourist destination. The shared path is good for inline skating.
Attractions	Experience plenty of fresh air and excellent views of Manhattan from the walkway high up in the bridge infrastructure.
Convenience	Start and finish at Clinton Street and Delancey Street in Manhattan, near the Delancey Street/ Essex Street subway station (F, J, M, and Z trains). Alternatively, start and/or finish at the Brooklyn end of the bridge, near the Marcy Avenue subway station (J, M, and Z trains).
Destination	If you finish this route at the Manhattan end, there are plenty of great pubs and restaurants nearby; see the route BR1 (Brooklyn and Manhattan Bridges) description for some ideas.

The Williamsburg Bridge connects Manhattan's Lower East Side to Brooklyn, roughly a mile upstream of the Manhattan Bridge. Opened in 1903, this suspension bridge was the second bridge built across the East River and, at that time, was the world's longest suspension bridge. This bridge is a popular commute route for cyclists and runners, and is also a popular out-and-back exercise route for on-footers working or living near its Manhattan end. While it carries heavy traffic and subway trains, it is blessed with pedestrian and bicycle paths up in the bridge superstructure, above the vehicle lanes and rail tracks.

There are two paths that pedestrians can use. Pedestrians and cyclists share the north side path, while the south side path is for pedestrians only. In describing this route, we assume an across-and-back outing, using one path out and the other one back. Since the two paths emerge at different places at the Brooklyn end, this involves a short connection via the streets at that end.

The ways to vary this route are obvious, starting and/or finishing at either end of the bridge.

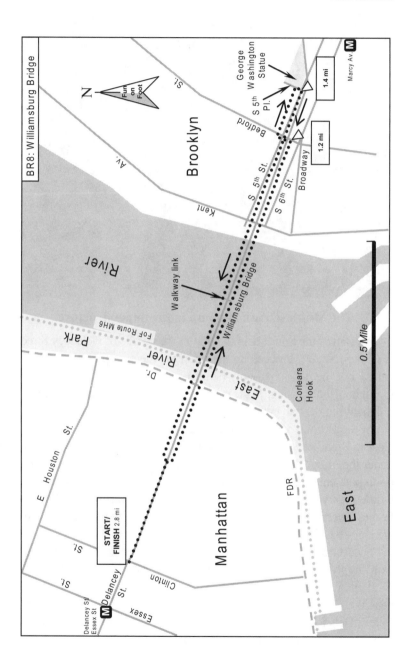

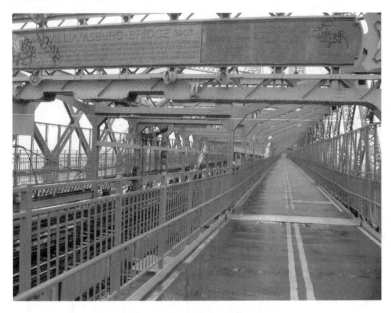

The Multiuse Path High up in the Superstructure

We start at the bridge access ramp in the middle of Delancey Street at Clinton Street. Proceed up the ramp to where it splits into the two paths. For the pedestrian-only (south) path go right. Enjoy the views throughout the crossing. In the middle of the bridge there is a connecting link between the two paths.

At the Brooklyn end, the south path emerges on Bedford Avenue, close to Broadway. To return on the north path, follow Bedford Avenue under the bridge and take the first right, following S 5th Street to the north path entrance ramp at S 5th Place. Across from this entrance is a little park with an equestrian statue of George Washington at Valley Forge. There are restrooms adjacent but when we were last there they were closed due to "sewer problems."

The Marcy Avenue subway station is a short walk from either path exit; simply follow the aboveground subway line to find that station.

If ending this walk on the Manhattan side, there are various eateries near the Delancey Street/Essex Street subway station. Better still, follow Delancey Street, Chrystie Street, and E Houston Street to our pub/restaurant suggestions of route BR1 (Brooklyn and Manhattan Bridges).

Marine Park

Distance	0.84 mile loop (Route BR9)
Comfort	Excellent running or walking conditions on a paved circuit around community sporting fields. Very popular on weekends and holidays, but the trails are wide enough for all comers. Good for inline skating on the inner circuit.
Attractions	A very pleasant community park.
Convenience	To get here you will probably drive. The alternative is to take the Q train to the Avenue U station and walk or take a bus east on Avenue U about a mile through a busy shopping area to the park.
Destination	No destination of note.

This is a large, attractive, popular park with many sporting fields and an encircling loop. The loop has two paved tracks. The inner track (0.81 mile) is for bikes and skates. The outer (0.84 mile) is for walkers and runners. The main parking area is at the south (Avenue U) end. There are restrooms at the north end.

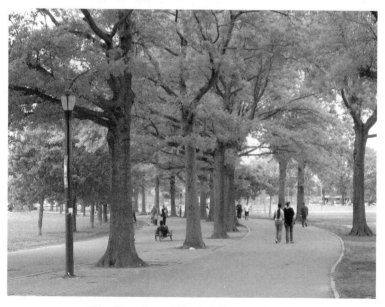

The Spacious Marine Park Circuit

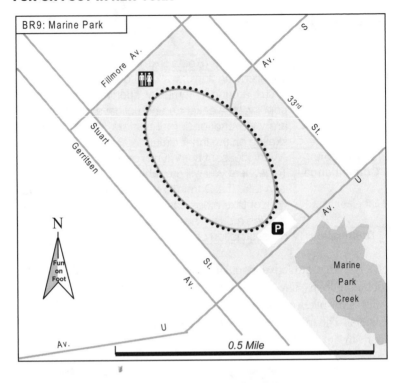

To get here you would probably either live nearby or drive. You can walk or get a bus down Avenue U from the subway. Avenue U is not a good running route since it is so busy with shops and small commercial establishments. There are plenty of food joints around here but no good pubs.

Other Routes

See the website of the Brooklyn Road Runners (www. brooklynroadrunners.org) for other suggested measured training routes in and near Prospect Park.

There are plans for a future greenway that will extend from Bay Ridge to Greenpoint, along the water. Watch for developments on that front.

Running Clubs

Brooklyn Queens Excel (groups.yahoo.com/group/bqe)
This is an all women's running team based in Brooklyn. It has both competitive and non-competitive runners united by a passion for running. The team provides strong support for each individual's running goals and meets in groups for regular runs. Everyone is invited to join in a morning run in Prospect Park on the first Saturday of every month. Meet at 8:00 am at Grand Army Plaza.
Email: crews.n@verizon.net

Brooklyn Road Runners Club (www.brooklynroadrunners.org)
Brooklyn Road Runners Club is a group of running buddies that meets mostly in Prospect Park. The club targets people who run for fun plus more serious athletes. "Everybody is welcome—if you feel you are a Brooklyn Road Runner, you probably are one." The club offers a bus to the marathon start, and hosts several races throughout the year, including races in Prospect Park and cross-country runs. There are regular group training runs four times a week, on Tuesday and Thursday evenings at 6:45 pm and Saturday and Sunday mornings at 9:00 am. There are monthly meetings at Knights of Columbus Hall on 10th Avenue near Prospect Park Southwest. See the website for more details.
Email: john_shostrom@simail.com

Club Atletico Mexicano de Neuva York (www.camny.org)
A club of about 85 members, predominantly Mexican but all nationalities are welcome. The club welcomes recreational and competitive runners and families, and meets regularly in Prospect Park.
Email: Refer to website

Prospect Park Track Club (www.pptc.org)
This club was founded over 30 years ago by Harry Murphy and a group of local runners. It has a proud tradition of spawning and preserving local running throughout the borough. Activities include Harry's Handicap (January 1), awards dinner (3rd Saturday in January), picnic and relay (June), bus to the New York City Marathon start, post-Marathon reception, monthly meetings, and monthly newsletters. Training includes coached speed sessions and weekend group runs. Events include the Cherry Tree 10 Miler (February), Al Goldstein

Speed Series (six 5K races Wednesday nights May-August), and The Turkey Trot 5 Miler on Thanksgiving Day.
Email: contact@pptc.org

Shore Road Striders (shoreroadstriders.org)
The Shore Road Striders Running Club is a running club for those individuals interested in running as a sport. Most of its runners come from the Bay Ridge neighborhood but membership is not limited to any one area. Meetings are held bimonthly and group runs are held almost every weekend starting at the 69th Street pier. Members enjoy each others' company on and off the running path.
Email: shoreroadstrid@aol.com

4

Queens

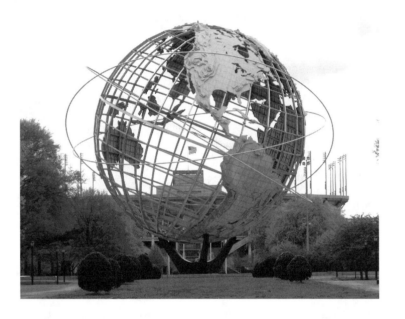

With a land area of 109 square miles, Queens is New York City's largest borough. It occupies the northwest corner of Long Island, abutting Brooklyn to the southwest and Nassau County to the east. It has a population of 2.2 million, a little smaller than Brooklyn's. The region was initially owned by the Dutch but attracted many English settlers. In the mid-17th century it came under English rule. Queens County was founded in 1683, and the region became a borough of New York City in 1898.[1]

Queens is an extremely diverse borough, with districts ranging from run-down industrial graveyards to classy high-end residential

---

1   Chapter head photo: The Unisphere in Flushing Meadows Corona Park.

enclaves. It is home to the city's two major airports, La Guardia and John F. Kennedy International. There are clusters of hotels around both airports, but not many elsewhere in the borough. The western part of the borough is well served by the subway network, but not so the eastern part where automobile travel is essential to living.

For the on-foot exerciser, there are some outstanding exercise routes, mostly associated with several large, green parks. We are featuring 12 Queens routes, including one extending into Manhattan and one extending into Brooklyn. Some routes are directly accessible by subway; the remainder by bus connections from subway stations.

Route	Distance
QN1 Queensboro-Triborough Bridges Loop	8.7 miles loop
QN2 Forest Park West	2.2 miles loop
QN3 Forest Park East	2.6 miles one way
QN4 Meadow Lake	3.7 miles loop
QN5 Flushing Meadows Corona Park	2.5 miles loop
QN6 Flushing Bay Promenade	2.6 miles out/back
QN7 Kissena Park	Various
QN8 The Motor Parkway	4.8 miles out/back
QN9 Alley Pond Park to Bayside	3.2 miles one way
QN10 Joe Michaels Mile	3.1 miles one way
QN11 Rockaway Beach Boardwalk	5.8 miles one way
QN12 Rockaway Park to Brooklyn	5.3 miles one way

These routes can be linked to each other in many different ways to form longer routes. Some possibilities are:

- Starting at the 75th Avenue subway station on Queens Boulevard, reverse route QN3 (Forest Park East), do route QN2 (Forest Park West), and return to the start via route QN3; total loop distance 7.4 miles;
- Starting at the park house in Forest Park, do route QN3 (Forest Park East) and then route QN4 (Meadow Lake), and return to the start by reversing route QN3; total loop distance 8.9 miles;
- Starting at the southeast corner of Alley Pond Park, link routes QN9 (Alley Pond Park to Bayside) and QN10 (Joe Michaels Mile) and finish at Fort Totten; total distance 5.2 miles one way;

- Starting at the Far Rockaway subway station, link routes QN11 (Rockaway Beach Boardwalk), QN12 (Rockaway Park to Brooklyn), and BR7 (Canarsie to Sheepshead Bay) to finish at the Sheepshead Bay subway station; total distance 13.8 miles one way.

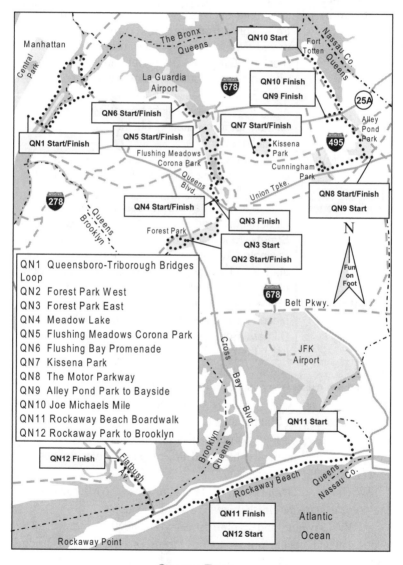

QN1 Queensboro-Triborough Bridges Loop
QN2 Forest Park West
QN3 Forest Park East
QN4 Meadow Lake
QN5 Flushing Meadows Corona Park
QN6 Flushing Bay Promenade
QN7 Kissena Park
QN8 The Motor Parkway
QN9 Alley Pond Park to Bayside
QN10 Joe Michaels Mile
QN11 Rockaway Beach Boardwalk
QN12 Rockaway Park to Brooklyn

Queens Routes

Queensboro-Triborough Bridges Loop

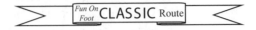

Distance	8.7 miles loop (Route QN1)
Comfort	This route involves 2.7 miles on excellent multiuse trails high up on bridges, 3.0 miles on a good, paved riverside trail, and 3.0 miles along streets, mostly in Queens. The street part is unattractive and uninspiring but the other parts make up for that. Expect to pass other on-footers everywhere along the route in daylight hours. Most parts are suitable for inline skating, but the street segments are quite rough.
Attractions	An exhilarating route with plenty of fresh air, some great city views, and very few interruptions by automobile traffic.
Convenience	Start and finish at the pedestrian ramp onto the Queensboro Bridge at First Avenue and E 60th Street in Manhattan, close to the subway station at Lexington Avenue and E 59th Street. Alternatively, start or end at any of several other subway stations close to the route in Manhattan or Queens.
Destination	There are several wind-down food and beverage places near our nominal finish point, and also in Ditmars Boulevard in Queens if you choose to finish there.

Our first route uses two East River bridges combined with trail segments in Manhattan and Queens. It is an excellent exercise loop for anyone living or staying on Manhattan's Upper East Side, northeast Midtown, or the Ravenswood or Astoria districts in Queens. It involves some invigorating trail segments above and along the East River and has very few cross-traffic encounters.[2]

We chose to start and finish in Manhattan, closest to Midtown hotels, but you can start and finish anywhere along the loop.

At First Avenue and E 60th Street you find the entrance to the pedestrian and bicycle ramp onto the Queensboro Bridge. This bridge, also known as the 59th Street Bridge, was opened in 1909.

2   Thanks to Jared Mestre for bringing this route to our attention.

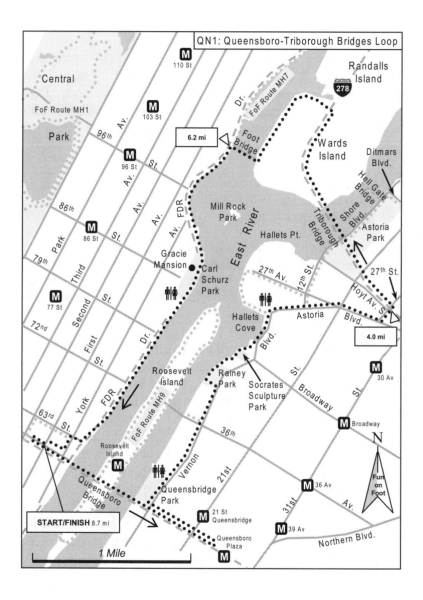

QN1: Queensboro-Triborough Bridges Loop

Randalls Island

Central

FoF Route MH1

110 St

FoF Route MH7

278

Park

103 St

96th

Av.

96 St

St.

6.2 mi

Foot Bridge

Wards Island

Ditmars Blvd.

86th

Av.

Av.

Av.

FDR

Mill Rock Park

East River

Hallets Pt.

Hell Gate Bridge

Shore Blvd.

Astoria Park

86 St

St.

Park

Third

79th

Gracie Mansion

Carl Schurz Park

Triborough Bridge

Hallets Cove

27th Av.

12th St.

27th St.

77 St

Second St.

72nd

First St.

Hoyt Av. S.

Astoria

Blvd.

4.0 mi

63rd St.

York

FDR

Dr.

Roosevelt Island

FoF Route MH9

Rainey Park

Socrates Sculpture Park

Blvd.

St.

Broadway

30 Av

Broadway

N

36th

Vernon

21st

Fun on Foot

Roosevelt Island

Queensboro Bridge

Queensbridge Park

21 St Queensbridge

31st

36 Av

Av.

START/FINISH 8.7 mi

Queensboro Plaza

39 Av

Northern Blvd.

1 Mile

Go up the ramp and across the bridge. Nobody would describe this as a beautiful experience—there is considerable vehicle noise and trains run above the pedestrian level. However, it is an excellent workout with loads of fresh air and no stops for traffic. You pass over Roosevelt Island (but there is no way down to there).

At the Queens end of the bridge walkway, swing 180 degrees back along the sidewalk to 21st Street. A nice shaded vehicle-free walkway starts here, taking you to Vernon Boulevard and Queensbridge Park. Turn right along the edge of the park. (There are restrooms at its northeast corner.) Continue on the Vernon Boulevard sidewalk to and past the power station, to the traffic signal at 36th Avenue.

VARIATION

You can go left on 36th Avenue across the Roosevelt Island Bridge to Roosevelt Island, where you can do an excellent on-foot loop. See the Manhattan route MH9 (Roosevelt Island) description for details. The bridge walkway gives access to level four of the main Roosevelt Island parking structure. Take the stairs or elevator to ground level to find the trails. After doing a loop here, you can get back to Manhattan via the tramway or to Manhattan or Queens via the subway F-train.

Proceed north up Vernon Boulevard, past the electric supply substation. This is not an attractive area. However, after 35th Avenue you come to Rainey Park, where you can track to the riverbank and follow a lovely paved trail. Rainey Park ends at the start of the Costco complex. Here the paved riverside trail continues behind the Costco buildings. You then come to the Socrates Sculpture Park. When we were last there, the park was under reconstruction but, by the time you read this, we hope you can proceed from Costco directly through that park (subject to cultural programs in progress at the time).

You then reconnect with the sidewalk of Vernon Boulevard. Continue for a few short blocks, through another quite unattractive industrial area. You then come to the Hallets Cove residential towers. There are restrooms on the street corner.

VARIATION

A riverside trail heads off to the left here. You can follow it around the Hallets Cove buildings to 27th Avenue. There is no point going further since it leads only to a very depressing industrial area. Follow 27th Avenue to 12th Street or on to Astoria Avenue to resume our main route.

From Hallets Cove, follow Main Avenue around into Astoria Boulevard. Continue to 12th Street.

VARIATION

To end your outing in Ditmars, Queens, follow 12th Street to the riverfront where it leads into Shore Boulevard. Go straight ahead along that street to a very pleasant trail that follows the river the length of beautiful Astoria Park. Expect plenty of other outdoor exercisers around here. Go under the Triborough Bridge and past the WWI monument. Continue under the Hell Gate rail bridge and take the first street heading inland, Ditmars Boulevard. Follow the sidewalk of Ditmars Boulevard several blocks through a mainly residential area.

At 31st Street there is a small commercial area, with several restaurants, predominantly Italian in cuisine. There is a subway station here (the terminus of the N and W lines, serving Midtown and Downtown Manhattan). If you want to end your outing with a beverage and a pub meal, continue on Ditmars Boulevard to 36th Street where you find McCann's Pub and Grill.

To continue back to Manhattan via the Triborough Bridge, follow Astoria Boulevard to 27th Street. Go left, cross Hoyt Avenue, and go under the bridge approach. Turn immediately right to the steps up to the walkway along the north side of the bridge.

The Triborough Bridge is actually more than a bridge—it is a set of bridges, highways, and viaducts that connect the boroughs of Manhattan, Queens, and the Bronx. The part that we feature is the East River suspension bridge, connecting Queens and Randall's Island.

The bridge walkway is good for pedestrians and is being continually improved. At the start of the cable span the walkway moves up to a level about 10 feet above the vehicle traffic and away to the right. This makes it a quite pleasant run or walk, despite the heavy road traffic nearby. Enjoy the fresh air in this crossing.

While on the bridge, look across the river to the Ward's Island footbridge and check that it is not in its raised position. You do not want to get to Ward's Island and have no way to continue to Manhattan.

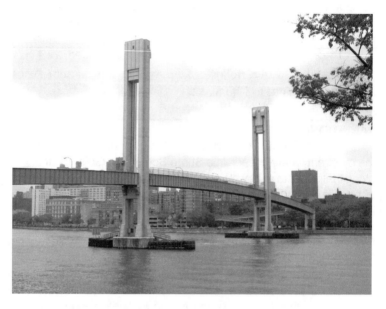

The Ward's Island East River Footbridge

At the Ward's Island end of the suspension bridge, the walkway peels off in a caged enclosure down to ground level. Ward's Island and Randall's Island were once separate islands but are now the one land mass, with Ward's Island to the south and Randall's Island to the north. Randall's Island hosts a stadium and other sporting facilities. Ward's Island has historically hosted more mundane city functions, but parts of it are being progressively converted into parkland.

As that construction progresses, on-foot options for negotiating Ward's Island will change. Our current recommendation is to proceed to the end of the pedestrian ramp and keep heading north, past the community institution buildings. Then go around to the left before the inlet that separates Ward's Island from the Randall's Island stadium. Pick up the paved trail south along the Manhattan side of Ward's Island. This trail leads to the footbridge, which delivers you to Manhattan on the East River trail at E 103rd Street.

Follow the trail down the East River, along the edge of busy Franklin D. Roosevelt Drive. At E 90th Street you reach Carl Schurz Park, where you escape from the highway and move to a pleasant pedestrian environment. Pass Gracie Mansion, the mayor's official residence. There are restrooms in Carl Schurz Park.

Continue on the raised plaza to E 81st Street, where Franklin D. Roosevelt Drive re-emerges from its tunnel and you must go down the steps and follow it again. There are pedestrian access bridges to the river trail at E 78th Street and E 71st Street.

At E 63rd Street take the ramp and crossover to York Avenue. Negotiate the streets to E 60th Street and First Avenue, where this route started.

There are innumerable bars and restaurants near here, if you want to wind down with a beverage or meal. Check out First, Second, and Third Avenues.

Forest Park West

Distance	2.2 miles loop (Route QN2)
Comfort	This route involves a 2.0-mile loop on a paved park trail, with a 0.1-mile connector from the start point. Motor vehicle traffic is not generally a concern. Expect plenty of other people around. It is mostly suitable for inline skating, but be prepared for a few rough patches.
Attractions	A pleasant exercise loop on a good quality trail.
Convenience	Start at the park house on Woodhaven Boulevard. There is a parking lot in Forest Park west of Woodhaven Boulevard. To get here by subway, take the J train to the 85th Street/Forest Parkway station. It is then 0.4 mile on a good street sidewalk to connect with the loop near the golf house.
Destination	There is no compelling destination, but there are other routes to link onto and plenty of beautiful parkland to enjoy around here.

Forest Park is an outstanding resource for Queens on-foot exercisers. It offers a variety of exercise routes, including paved trails and earth trails. The park is tucked into a southwest corner of Queens, near the Brooklyn line. It is one Queens park that can be conveniently reached by subway.

For this book, we have split Forest Park into two parts. This first route description covers the park west of Woodhaven Boulevard. This is the less exciting side for on-foot exercisers, but it does have a good exercise loop. Furthermore, you can easily add this loop onto routes based on the east side of the park, possibly extending as far as Flushing Bay—the following route descriptions explain this.

We nominally start at the park house at the intersection of Forest Park Drive and Woodhaven Boulevard. There is a small ranger station here where you can pick up a trail map. Follow Forest Park Drive past the 1904 carousel on your right. Continue on either of the side trails along the drive. They are pleasant and traffic is usually light. Continue to the entrance to the golf course. Snacks and restrooms are available at the golf house.

Go left along the paved road that today is no more than a parking lot. Follow the road to its end barrier, at Forest Parkway. At this point, a

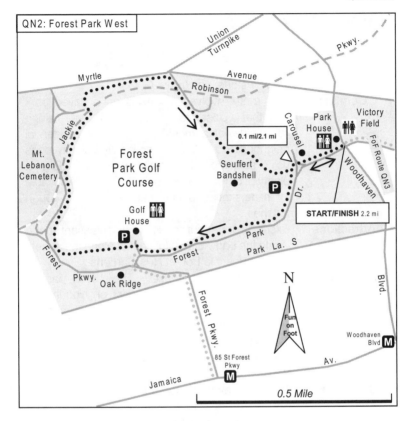

nice new paved multiuse trail starts up. Follow it around the edge of the golf course and eventually under the Jackie Robinson Parkway. Bear right on the paved trail between the parkway and Myrtle Avenue.

Continue to the next intersection where there is a road going to the right under the parkway. It is primarily a highway ramp but it also leads to a closed road heading back into Forest Park, around the golf course boundary. At the end of the paved road, there is a short unpaved path to the Seuffert Bandshell and the adjacent parking area. The bandshell is named for George Seuffert, Sr. whose band started a tradition of Sunday concerts in the park in 1905. Go through the parking area, back to the trafficked roads near the carousel. Retrace your original steps on Forest Park Drive, back to the park house and Woodhaven Boulevard.

Forest Park East

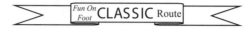

Distance	2.6 miles one way (route QN3)
Comfort	This route involves 1.4 miles on a paved park road that is closed to vehicles plus 1.2 miles along street sidewalks, mostly in an upscale residential neighborhood. You can optionally build in loops using soft, wide bridle trails in the park. Expect plenty of other people around. It is mostly suitable for inline skating, but be prepared for a few rough patches.
Attractions	Excellent underfoot conditions and pleasant shade inside the park. Beautiful homes along the streets through upscale Forest Hills Gardens.
Convenience	Start at the park house. There is a parking lot nearby, in Forest Park west of Woodhaven Boulevard. It is roughly a half-mile to the nearest subway station at Woodhaven Boulevard and Jamaica Avenue (J and Z lines). Finish at the 75th Avenue subway station (E and F lines) on Queens Boulevard.
Destination	There are several restaurants and bars on Queens Boulevard, for a food or beverage break before catching a subway home.

The east side of Forest Park has a variety of excellent on-foot exercise paths, including a rubberized running circuit, paved trails, soft earth trails, and some more-challenging hiking trails. The gem is the paved road, Forest Park Drive, now permanently closed to motor vehicles for almost 1.4 miles. We chose to feature the latter as our primary route, but many variations are possible.

Start at the park house at the intersection of Forest Park Drive and Woodhaven Boulevard. There is a small ranger station here where you can pick up a trail map. Cross Woodhaven Boulevard and follow Forest Park Drive through the vehicle barrier and along the edge of Victory Field. There is an excellent 400-meter running track here.

Continue across the overpasses over the disused rail tracks and Myrtle Avenue. After the latter, on the left is a trailhead to the network of hiking trails. There are three hiking trails (not shown on our map):

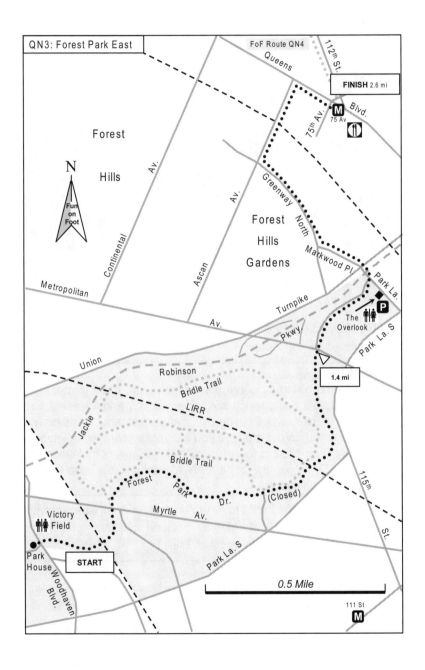

QN3: Forest Park East

FoF Route QN4
Queens

112th St.

FINISH 2.6 mi

Forest

Blvd.

75th Av.

M 75 Av

N

Fun
on
Foot

Hills

Av.

Greenway

Av.

North

Forest

Hills

Markwood Pl.

Gardens

Continental

Ascan

Park La.

P

Metropolitan

Turnpike

The
Overlook

Av.

Park La. S

Pkwy.

1.4 mi

Union

Robinson

Bridle Trail

LIRR

115th

Jackie

Bridle Trail

Forest

Park

Dr.

(Closed)

St.

Victory
Field

Myrtle

Av.

Park

Dr.

(Closed)

Park La. S

START

0.5 Mile

Park
House

Woodhaven

Blvd.

111 St

M

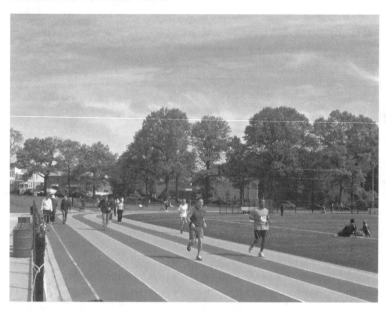

The Popular Victory Field Running Track

the blue-blazed 1.7-mile loop, the orange-blazed 2.4-mile loop, and the yellow-blazed 1.0-mile loop.

VARIATION

While the hiking trails are somewhat rough, there is also the network of bridle trails, which are wide and soft and excellent for running. (Stay well away from horses, if any are present.) The bridle trails are marked on our map, so you can make your own trail loop. The Forest Park Classic four-mile race employs a combination of Forest Park Drive and the bridle trails, finishing with a loop of the Victory Field running track.

Continue on Forest Park Drive to the road junction with sporting fields and a picnic area to the right. This road spur takes you to the intersection of Myrtle Avenue and Park Lane S.

VARIATION

Another variation that you can use to create loop routes in the east side of Forest Park is the sidewalk of Park Lane S, which is pleasant and shady and has no cross-traffic intersections.

Cross over the rail tracks and continue to Metropolitan Avenue. After this point, Forest Park Drive is again open to vehicles. Cross

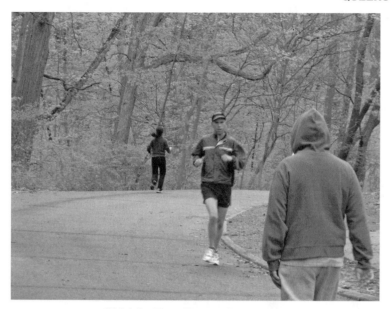

Vehicle-Free Forest Park Drive

Metropolitan Avenue and follow the sidewalk of Forest Park Drive to the park boundary. At the park entrance is The Overlook, an imposing building now managed by the parks department.

We have chosen to now lead you to Queens Boulevard, for three reasons. First, there are restaurants, bars, and a subway station, so it is a good place to finish a route. Second, the route through the streets is very attractive, passing through a beautiful residential neighborhood. Third, this is the main connecting route to Flushing Meadows Corona Park, allowing you to string together more routes in this part of Queens.

Exit the park on Park Lane, near where several busy roads converge. Go left over Jackie Robinson Parkway and cross Union Turnpike. Then follow Markwood Place into the lovely residential neighborhood of Forest Hills Gardens. Turn right into Greenway North and follow it to Ascan Avenue. Turn right there and continue across the rail tracks to busy, extra-wide Queens Boulevard.[3]

Turn right and proceed to the subway station at 75th Avenue. There are many eating places around here and a couple of good pubs. Nola and I enjoy having a beverage at Cobblestones, a block further along Queens Boulevard, before catching the train.

3   Thanks to Bonnie Harper for suggesting this part of the route.

Meadow Lake

Distance	3.7 miles loop (Route QN4)
Comfort	This route involves 0.8 mile each way from Queens Boulevard to the lake along street sidewalks, plus a 2.1-mile loop of the lake on a paved park trail. Expect plenty of other people around. It is mostly suitable for inline skating, but be prepared for a few rough patches.
Attractions	Excellent underfoot conditions and a very pleasant environment around the lake.
Convenience	Start and finish at the 75th Avenue subway station (E and F lines) on Queens Boulevard. You can connect with route QN3 (Forest Park East).
Destination	There are several restaurants and bars on Queens Boulevard, for a food or beverage break before catching a subway home.

Meadow Lake occupies the part of Flushing Meadows Corona Park south of the Long Island Expressway. While you can get to Meadow Lake from the main part of that park, you can also get to it from the vicinity of Forest Park. We chose to describe the latter approach, making it easy to connect a loop of Meadow Lake onto route QN3 (Forest Park East).[4]

Start where route QN3 finished, at 75th Avenue and Queens Boulevard, on the north side of Queens Boulevard. Follow 112th Street north to Jewell Avenue. Turn right and follow Jewell Avenue across Grand Central Parkway. You then need to cross the road to your left to enter the park near the south end of Meadow Lake. Be extra careful—there is no pedestrian crossing!

Go right for a counterclockwise loop of the lake. Pass the interestingly themed Triassic Playground, where there are restrooms. This is a very pleasant lake environment, with an abundance of birdlife and flowering trees. Proceed around the lake, past the model airplane field and boat and bike rental, to the kiosk at the north end of the lake.

---

4   Thanks to Bonnie Harper for bringing this combined route to our attention.

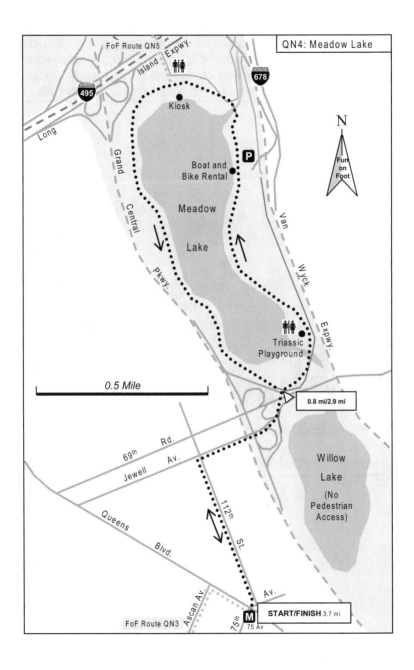

QN4: Meadow Lake

FoF Route QN5

Island Expwy.

Long

Grand

Central

Pkwy.

Kiosk

Boat and
Bike Rental

Meadow

Lake

N

Fun
on
Foot

Van

Wyck

Expwy.

Triassic
Playground

0.5 Mile

0.8 mi/2.9 mi

69th Rd.

Jewell Av.

Queens Blvd.

112th St.

Willow

Lake

(No
Pedestrian
Access)

Ascan Av.

75th

Av.

START/FINISH 3.7 mi

FoF Route QN3

75 Av

> **VARIATION**
> Immediately north of the kiosk is the wide pedestrian bridge over Long Island Expressway leading to the main part of Flushing Meadows Corona Park. Use this bridge to continue going north—see route QN5 (Flushing Meadows Corona Park) for more details. In fact you can link together the whole chain of routes QN2 through QN6.

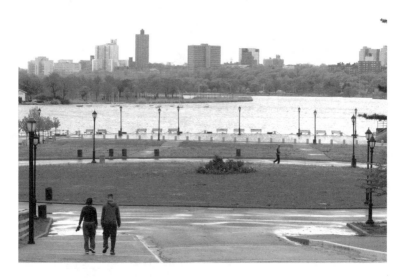

Meadow Lake Viewed from its North End

Continue around the lake to its south end and retrace your route back to the start point at Queens Boulevard.

Flushing Meadows Corona Park

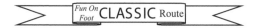

Distance	2.5 miles loop (Route QN5)
Comfort	This route involves paved park trails and vehicle-free roads throughout, with many possible variations. Expect plenty of other people around. There are ample opportunities for inline skating.
Attractions	An outstanding environment for on-foot exercise. Several relics from the 1964 New York World's Fair are still in place.
Convenience	Start and finish at the Willets Point subway station on the 7 line.
Destination	There are several interesting destinations here, including the Queens Museum of Art, Queens Wildlife Center, and Queens Botanical Garden. There are restaurants and bars about a half-mile away, west on Roosevelt Avenue.

Flushing Meadows Corona Park, the largest park in Queens, is well known to many sports fans as the location of Citi Field, home of the New York Mets, and the USTA Billie Jean King National Tennis Center. It is also the location of the Queens Museum of Art and the Queens Wildlife Center (Queens Zoo).

However, this park is much more than that. It is a truly fascinating place. The fascination stems from its origin as the site of the 1939 New York World's Fair and its later role as the venue of the 1964 New York World's Fair. Since the latter event concluded, time in the park has largely stood still. Most of the fair layout is still there, complete with roads, paths, pools, and fountains, plus some famous relics including the Unisphere, the scale model panorama of New York City in what is now the Queens Museum of Art, and the derelict Observatory Towers of the once-spectacular New York State Pavilion.

Most significantly, Flushing Meadows Corona Park today is an outstanding place for on-foot exercise. There are innumerable choices of running routes along the various paths and vehicle-free roads.

There are so many running route options within this park it is not practical for us to catalog them or recommend particular routes.

Consider the 2.5-mile route shown on the map as simply one illustrative example of what you might do, starting and ending at the Willets Point subway station in the park.

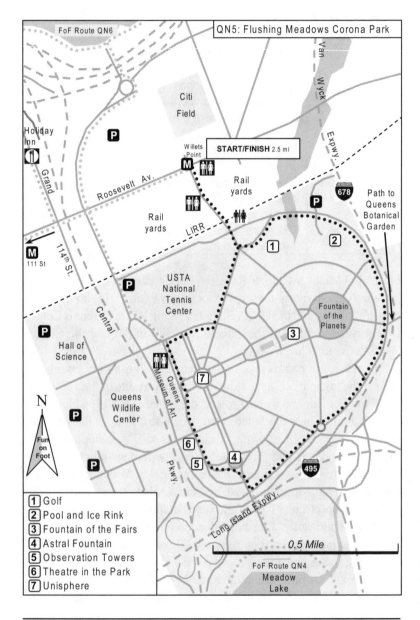

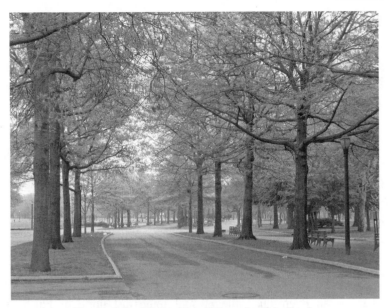

Typical On-Foot Conditions in this Park

Other options you might consider are:

- Connecting to Meadow Lake via the bridge over the Long Island Expressway; see route QN4 (Meadow Lake);
- Connecting to the Flushing Bay Promenade via the stadium parking area; see route QN6 (Flushing Bay Promenade); and
- Connecting to the Queens Botanical Garden via the path under the Van Wyck Expressway and over College Point Boulevard. Note however that the Botanical Garden is not well suited to running.

If you are interested in a food or beverage stop after your exercise, you need to leave the park. The best option is to go about a half-mile west along Roosevelt Avenue from the Willets Point subway station to the area around the 111th Street subway station. There are several food places and a basic pub here. For a better restaurant/bar experience, go up 114th Street to the La Guardia Holiday Inn where there is a good sports bar with excellent food.

Flushing Bay Promenade

Distance	2.6 miles out and back (Route QN6)
Comfort	This is an out-and-back route on a paved trail along the shore of Flushing Bay. Expect other company but crowds are unlikely. Good for inline skating.
Attractions	An excellent escape from the hustle of the La Guardia Airport district, with plenty of fresh air.
Convenience	Convenient to some La Guardia Airport hotels, including the Marriott and Crowne Plaza. Start and finish at the overpass from Ditmars Boulevard across Grand Central Parkway at 27th Avenue. Can also be accessed from the Willets Point subway station on the 7 line.
Destination	No specific destination.

There is an interesting little on-foot route just north of Flushing Meadows Corona Park, along the shore of Flushing Bay. What makes it most interesting is its proximity to La Guardia Airport hotels. Therefore, this is a route that every road warrior who ever stays near the airport should know.

Start at the overpass across the highway where 27th Avenue meets Ditmars Boulevard in East Elmhurst. This is roughly two blocks from the La Guardia Marriott and the Crowne Plaza. Cross the overpass to the start of the paved trail. Follow the trail around the shore, past the World's Fair Marina, to the trail's end after 1.3 miles. The views of the water make this a very pleasant outing. Retrace your steps to where you started.

The trail can also be accessed via an overpass at 31st Drive, close to the intersection of Astoria Boulevard and 108th Street, and via a street under the highway near the parking lots for Citi Field. The latter also connects to the Willets Point subway station and Flushing Meadows Corona Park.

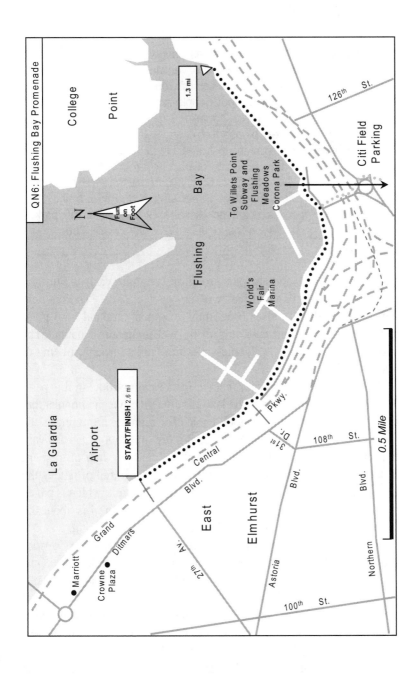

QN6: Flushing Bay Promenade

College Point

1.3 mi

Flushing Bay

To Willets Point Subway and Flushing Meadows Corona Park

N

Fun on Foot

Flushing

World's Fair Marina

Citi Field Parking

126th St.

La Guardia Airport

START/FINISH 2.6 mi

Pkwy.

Central Blvd.

31st Dr.

108th St.

0.5 Mile

Grand

Ditmars

Marriott

Crowne Plaza

27th Av.

East

Elmhurst

Blvd.

Blvd.

Astoria

Northern

100th St.

Kissena Park

Distance	Various (Route QN7)
Comfort	This route involves paved park trails and street sidewalks, with no vehicle crossings and many different choices of route variation. Expect plenty of other people around. There are ample opportunities for inline skating.
Attractions	A very pleasant parkland setting.
Convenience	Convenient to some La Guardia Airport hotels, There is plenty of parking around the park. To get to the park by public transit take the 7 train to Flushing Main Street station and then travel 1¼ miles south on Kissena Boulevard to the park, either on-foot or via a Q25, Q34, or Q17 bus.
Destination	No specific destination.

Kissena Park is a popular park, roughly one mile east of Flushing Meadows Corona Park. It has two very distinct parts. The northern half of the park comprises beautifully groomed parkland with trees, gardens, a picturesque lake, and many well maintained paths. The southern half is mostly wilderness, with the trails through it being of questionable quality.

There is no single obvious choice for a running route in this park. The trail around the edge of the lake is very attractive and popular, but only 0.5 mile in length. A good choice for runners in training is the perimeter sidewalk of the park, which is a 1.9-mile loop. One can vary that by using some of the paths through the northern half of the park instead of the northern perimeter sidewalk. A third trail of note is the east-west multiuse trail through the middle of the park, which is paved and considered part of the Greenway system. This trail is about 0.6 miles long and can be used to build a loop of your own liking.

West of Kissena Park is a narrow greenbelt, called Kissena Corridor West, which stretches for roughly a mile to the Queens Botanical Garden and the edge of Flushing Meadows Corona Park. You can negotiate Kissena Corridor West on foot.

On the eastern side of Kissena Park there is another greenbelt, called Kissena Corridor East, stretching roughly 1.5 miles to the northwest corner of Cunningham Park—see route QN8 (The Motor Parkway) for more details of that park. Kissena Corridor East mainly comprises sporting fields. It can be negotiated on foot, mostly along street sidewalks, and there are several roads to cross. That piece of greenbelt therefore is of limited appeal to the on-foot exerciser.

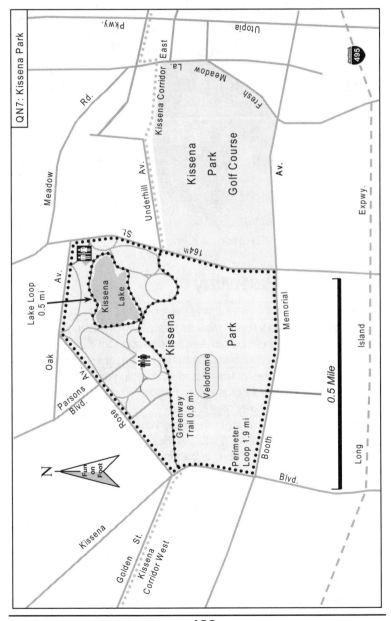

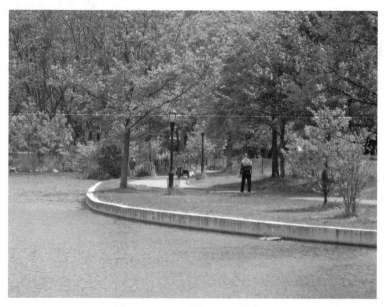

Picturesque Kissena Lake

The Motor Parkway

Distance	4.8 miles out and back (Route QN8)
Comfort	This route involves beautifully maintained, mostly shady, paved park trails throughout. Expect plenty of other people around. Good for inline skating.
Attractions	A very pleasant parkland setting and a trail with no vehicle crossings. Read the history of the Motor Parkway on the signs.
Convenience	Start and finish at the park house of Alley Pond Park on Winchester Boulevard near Union Turnpike. There is parking here. To get here (or to Cunningham Park) by public transit, take the E or F train to Kew Gardens Union Turnpike station and catch a Q46 bus along Union Turnpike.
Destination	In Alley Pond Park there are several other pleasant walking or running trails, and a scenic environment in which to relax.

The Motor Parkway is as exciting to historians as it is to on-foot exercisers. This two-mile stretch of paved multiuse trail is one of the few sections that remain of one of America's most historic roads. It was built by William K. Vanderbilt, Jr., great-grandson of railroad baron Cornelius Vanderbilt, beginning in 1908. When completed, it stretched 48 miles from Queens to Lake Ronkonkoma in Suffolk County. Operated as a privately owned toll road, it closed in 1938 when the business was no longer viable.

Today, this is a beautifully landscaped, shady trail linking Alley Pond Park and Cunningham Park in east Queens. It is very popular with runners and walkers and justifiably so.

The only obvious way to use this trail is as an out-and-back route, starting from either end. There is ample parking at both ends. We chose to start and finish in Alley Pond Park, at the park house on Winchester Boulevard. Alley Pond Park, with 635 acres, is the second largest park in Queens. The park house is home to the Alley Pond Striders, a very active and friendly local running and walking club.

From the park house, head immediately south, past the tennis courts, to the start of the Motor Parkway. Head west, go under the highway bridge, and keep following the straight path of the Motor Parkway.

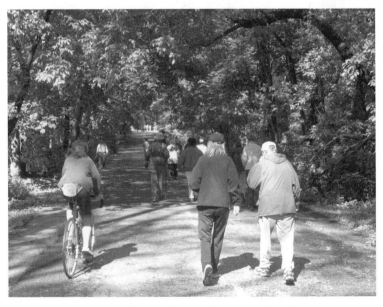

The Popular Motor Parkway Trail

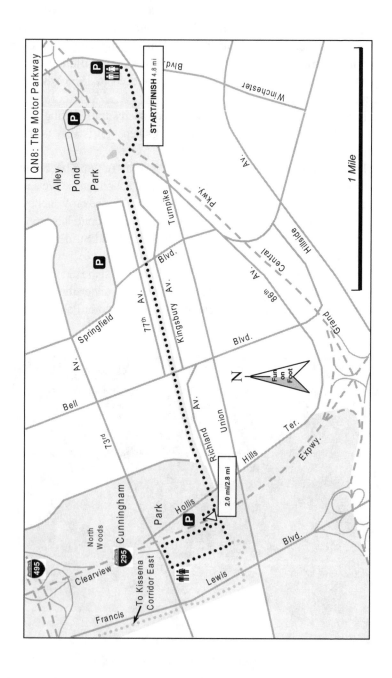

VARIATION

There are some pleasant forest trails in Alley Pond Park, accessed from the Motor Parkway by paths to the right after the highway bridge. The annual Alley Pond five-mile race uses a combination of these trails and the Motor Parkway.

Proceed on to Cunningham Park, appreciating the vehicle-free conditions, especially the overpass over busy Bell Boulevard. Eventually the pleasant environment comes to an end when you hit the ugly embankment of the Clearview Expressway in Cunningham Park. The two-mile marker of the Motor Parkway is right here.

Cunningham Park, with 358 acres of land, is a large park which provides mixed value to the local outdoor community. The northern part, known as the North Woods, is quite rugged and dedicated mainly to mountain bike trails. South of 73rd Avenue, there are open sporting fields. This is where the Motor Parkway delivers you.

We suggest a 0.8-mile loop of the sports fields on the west side of the Clearview Expressway, before going back to Alley Pond Park. To do this, turn right, heading north along the Clearview Expressway embankment to an underpass under the expressway. Across the highway you find the sporting fields. Do a loop around them, passing the restrooms at the northwest corner. Continue back to the Motor Parkway and retrace your steps to the start point.

VARIATION

Having crossed to the west side of the Clearview Expressway, you can follow the Greenway signs to connect to Kissena Corridor East and on to Kissena Park. See the route QN7 (Kissena Park) description for more information.

Alley Pond Park to Bayside

Distance	3.2 miles one way (Route QN9)
Comfort	The first 2.4 miles are on park trails, partly paved and partly earth. These are relatively little used trails. The final 0.8 mile is on street sidewalks. Not suitable for inline skating.
Attractions	Trails mostly in a pleasant parkland setting with few vehicle crossings. A very useful connection between the south part of Alley Pond Park and Little Neck Bay on Long Island Sound.
Convenience	Start at the park house of Alley Pond Park on Winchester Boulevard near Union Turnpike. To get here by public transit, take the E or F train to Kew Gardens Union Turnpike station and catch a Q46 bus along Union Turnpike. The route ends at the intersection of Northern Boulevard and Bell Boulevard. There is a Long Island Railroad station here, with service to Penn Station in Manhattan, or a Q12 or Q13 bus to Flushing Main Street subway station on the 7 line.
Destination	In Bayside there are several restaurants and bars to choose from for a wind-down food or beverage break. You can also connect to route QN10 (Joe Michaels Mile).

This route is particularly interesting because it provides a link from the south end of Alley Pond Park (and the Motor Parkway covered in route QN8) to the lively suburb of Bayside and Little Neck Bay on Long Island Sound. In Bayside you can connect to another excellent trail described as route QN10 (Joe Michaels Mile). Also in Bayside there is a train station plus restaurants and bars making for a great place to end a route.

We chose to describe this as a one-way route, ending in the lively part of Bayside, which works well if you don't mind taking public transit to and from your exercise route. However, there are many other ways to use this route, including out-and-back from either end, or combining it with route QN8 (The Motor Parkway) or QN10 (Joe Michaels Mile) for a quality longer route.

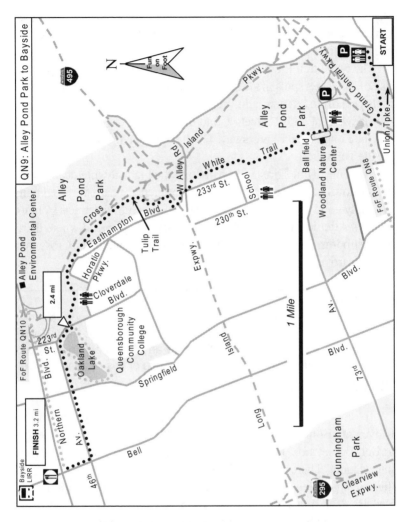

Start at the park house on Winchester Boulevard north of Union Turnpike and head immediately south, past the tennis courts, to the start of the Motor Parkway. Head west and go under the highway bridge. Take the first or second path to the right off the Motor Parkway. There are many paths here but, provided you head generally north, you will come to a large open area with a football field, other activities, and a restroom building at the south end.

Bear left past the Woodland Nature Center to the ball field. Follow the paved path around the ball field and watch carefully for the white-blazed trail, heading off north from the left outfield. There are other trails here as well and the blazing is not perfect, so be prepared to exercise a little patience.

The white trail is an earth trail and is ideal for running, except for a risk of some wet spots in the spring. Continue to its northern end where trails peel off to left and right. Take the left path, which delivers you to the sidewalk of 233rd Street. Go to the right and cross W Alley Road and the Long Island Expressway. On the right you find a new trailhead, for the Tulip Trail.

The Tulip Trail skirts a jug-handle of the highway interchange and then follows the Cross Island Parkway north. It is a narrow paved trail, generally good but the proximity of the highway traffic detracts from its quality. After leaving the highway, it passes a playground where there are restrooms. It then emerges on Cloverdale Boulevard. Cross that street to arrive at the edge of pretty Oakland Lake.

VARIATION

There is a pleasant 0.7-mile paved loop trail around Oakland Lake. If you are doing an out-and-back route from the Alley Pond Park house, we suggest doing this loop and then backtracking on the Tulip Trail and White Trail. Total distance of this route would be 5.5 miles.

To continue on to the Bayside restaurant area, go north on Cloverdale Boulevard to 46th Avenue and follow that street to the left to Bell Boulevard. Turn right and proceed to the Northern Boulevard intersection. There are several restaurants and bars to choose from on this stretch of Bell Boulevard. The Long Island Railroad station is on Bell Boulevard, a little north of Northern Boulevard. The buses to Flushing Main Street subway station run on Northern Boulevard.

VARIATION

To continue directly on to route QN10 (Joe Michaels Mile) you do not need to go to Bell Boulevard. From Oakland Lake, go north on 223rd Street to Northern Boulevard to intersect that route.

Joe Michaels Mile

Distance	3.1 miles one way (Route QN10)
Comfort	The first 2.4 miles are on a paved multiuse trail. The final 0.7 mile is on street sidewalks. Expect plenty of other people around. The multiuse trail is good for inline skating.
Attractions	An excellent quality trail for 2.4 miles with no vehicle crossings and some scenic views over Little Neck Bay.
Convenience	Start at the entrance to Fort Totten near 212th Street and Bell Boulevard. There is parking here. To get here by public transit, take the 7 train to Flushing Main Street station and catch a Q13 or Q16 bus to Fort Totten. The route ends at the intersection of Northern Boulevard and Bell Boulevard. There is a Long Island Railroad station here, with service to Penn Station in Manhattan, or a Q12 or Q13 bus to Flushing Main Street subway station.
Destination	In Bayside there are several restaurants and bars to choose from for a wind-down food or beverage break. You can also connect to route QN9 (Alley Pond Park to Bayside).

Joe Michaels Mile is a paved multiuse trail along the shore of Little Neck Bay between the north end of Alley Pond Park and the Fort Totten reservation on Willets Point. It is named in memory of Joseph Michaels (1941-87), a local fitness activist, marathon runner, and first president of the Alley Pond Striders running club.

This 2.4-mile trail is popular with local runners, walkers, and cyclists. They typically go out and back, starting from either end. We chose to describe it one way, starting from the Fort Totten end where there is more parking. We tack another 0.7 mile onto the south end to finish at the same lively restaurant and bar area as route QN9 (Alley Pond Park to Bayside). There is a bus service along Bell Boulevard (bus Q13) connecting start and finish, should you need that.

Start at the entrance to Fort Totten reservation, where you find the trailhead for Joe Michaels Mile. The trail is sandwiched between the shore of Little Neck Bay and the busy Cross Island Parkway. Go for 2.4 miles on this uninterrupted, paved trail. The biggest downside of this

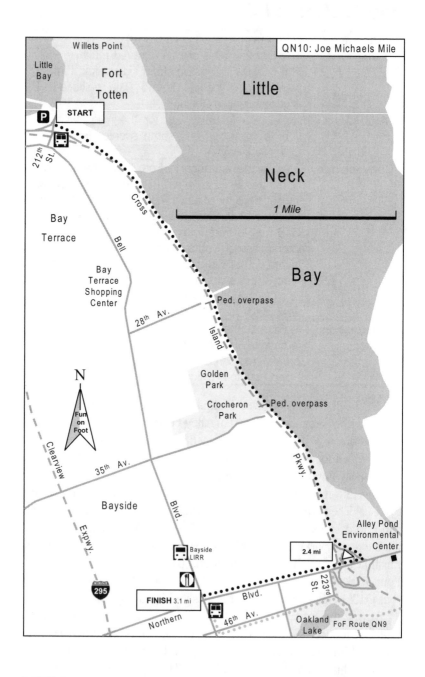

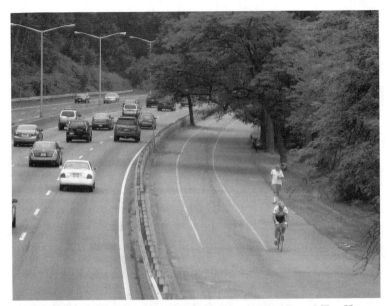

Joe Michaels Mile and the Accompanying Road Traffic

trail is the proximity of the parkway traffic. However, the open water on the other side alleviates the unpleasantness to some extent.

There are two pedestrian overpasses from the trail over the parkway to residential Bayside—one at 28th Avenue and one at 35th Avenue (Crocheron Park).

The trail ends at Northern Boulevard, immediately east of the parkway interchange. Using the sidewalk, head west to the Bell Boulevard intersection. There are restaurants, bars, and buses here. The Long Island Railroad station is north up Bell Boulevard.

VARIATION

You can connect this route and route QN9 (Alley Pond Park to Bayside), using 223rd Street to go between Oakland Lake and Northern Boulevard. The resultant distance between Fort Totten and the southeast corner of Alley Pond Park is 5.2 miles.

As another alternative, across Northern Boulevard from the Joe Michaels Mile trailhead is the Alley Pond Environmental Center and its own network of trails in the northern part of Alley Pond Park. It is possible to use those trails to connect through to the south end of Alley Pond Park. However, this is very low-lying land and these trails can be very questionable for outdoor exercise purposes.

Rockaway Beach Boardwalk

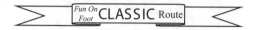

Distance	5.8 miles one way (Route QN11)
Comfort	4.7 miles are on the boardwalk, which is wide and level. The other 1.1 miles are on street sidewalks. Expect other people around, with possible crowding in spots on a summer weekend day. Not recommended for inline skating, which is prohibited from 10:00 am to 6:00 pm anyway.
Attractions	A beautiful beach environment with no vehicles, no dogs, and no bicycles between 10:00 am and 6:00 pm.
Convenience	Start at the Far Rockaway subway station and finish at the Rockaway Park subway station, both on the A line. There are several other subway stations between these two ends so you can easily get to and from intermediate points as well.
Destination	At Rockaway Park there are restaurants and bars for wind-down food or beverage, plus a beautiful beach for relaxing.

Rockaway Beach is a quite amazing part of New York City. It is a long ocean beach, with surfing, bathing, and everything else a good beach has to offer. It has a boardwalk, a little over five miles long, stretching from Beach 9th Street to Beach 126th Street. The boardwalk is reachable from subway stations at several points. Dogs are prohibited from May 1 to October 1 and bikes are prohibited from 10:00 am to 6:00 pm.

We chose to start at the east end and finish close to the west end. One downside of this routing is that you have to travel almost a mile on street sidewalks to get from the Far Rockaway station to the boardwalk. Therefore, you might prefer to start from the Beach 25th Street or Beach 36th Street subway station instead, both being significantly closer to the beach.

If starting from the Far Rockaway subway station, follow Mott Avenue east to its end at Beach 13th Street. Then keep going straight ahead to link to Beach 9th Street. Go right here and follow Beach 9th Street down to the start of the boardwalk.

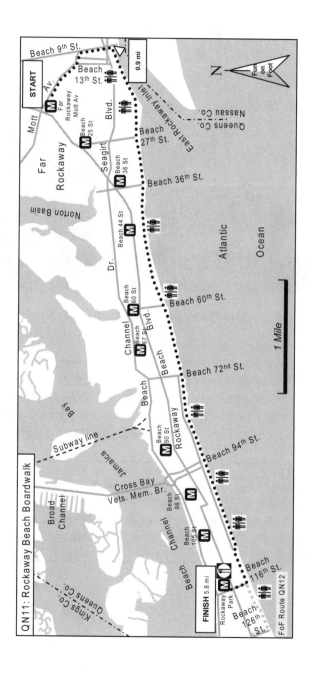

QN11: Rockaway Beach Boardwalk

START

Beach 9th St.

Beach 13th St.

Far Rockaway Mott Av

Mott Av.

Far Rockaway

Seagirt Blvd.

Beach 25 St

Beach 36 St

Norton Basin

Beach 44 St

Channel Dr.

Beach 60 St

Beach 67 St.

Channel Blvd.

Jamaica Bay

Beach Rockaway

Subway line

Beach 90 St

Cross Bay Vets. Mem. Br.

Broad Channel

Beach 98 St

Beach 105 St

Beach Channel

FINISH 5.8 mi

Rockaway Park

Beach 126th St.

FoF Route QN12

East Rockaway Inlet

0.9 mi

N

Fun on Foot

Queens Co.
Nassau Co.

Beach 27th St.

Beach 36th St.

Beach 60th St.

Beach 72nd St.

Atlantic Ocean

1 Mile

Beach 94th St.

Beach 116th St.

Kings Co.
Queens Co.

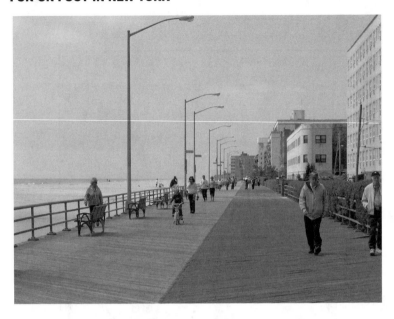

The Wide, Popular Boardwalk

There are several restrooms along the boardwalk, open seasonally.

Continue to Beach 116th Street in Rockaway Park. The boardwalk continues for another half-mile but this is the most convenient place to leave it to get to the last subway station. Go inland up Beach 116th Street to Rockaway Beach Boulevard. There are restaurants and bars here and the subway station is a little further up Beach 116th Street.

VARIATION

You can also connect to route QN12 (Rockaway Park to Brooklyn) here, to get to Brooklyn. To do so, simply continue along the boardwalk at Beach 116th Street, instead of turning inland to the subway station. If doing that, subtract 0.4 mile from the sum of the two route distances.

Rockaway Park to Brooklyn

Distance	5.3 miles one way (Route QN12)
Comfort	The first 3.2 miles in the Rockaways are roughly half on beach boardwalks and half on good street sidewalks. The remainder of the route is on a paved trail running adjacent to a busy road. While there is a lot of traffic nearby, there is also considerable fresh sea air. Expect other people around, more cyclists than pedestrians. Not recommended overall for inline skating, but sections of the route are good for that.
Attractions	A route with long stretches close to the sea and few vehicle intersections to slow you down.
Convenience	Start at the Rockaway Park subway station, on the A line, or connect from other Rockaway Beach locations via the boardwalk. Finish where Flatbush Avenue intersects the Belt Parkway. From here, follow route BR7 (Canarsie to Sheepshead Bay) to the Sheepshead Bay subway station, for a total distance of 8.4 miles.
Destination	Sheepshead Bay is a lively center with various pubs and restaurants and convenient subway access back to the main centers. You can alternatively continue on-foot a short distance along the sidewalks to Brighton Beach or Coney Island.

If you are seeking a longer route with excellent running conditions, this can be an ideal outing. You need to combine it with Brooklyn route BR7 (Canarsie to Sheepshead Bay) to give the full subway-to-subway route with a distance of 8.4 miles. It is also easy to tack on further distance of up to 5.4 additional miles using route QN11 (Rockaway Beach Boardwalk).

Start at the Rockaway Park subway station near Rockaway Beach Boulevard and Beach 116th Street. Go down the latter street to the sea to join the Rockaway Beach boardwalk and head to the right.

Continue to the end of the boardwalk at Beach 126th Street. Head inland to Rockaway Beach Boulevard and turn left there. Follow the sidewalk for roughly a mile through a pleasant residential area.

At Beach 149th Street enter Jacob Riis Park. Continue straight ahead and then take the first path to the left to join the boardwalk that starts there. Follow the boardwalk past the beach pavilion to its western end.

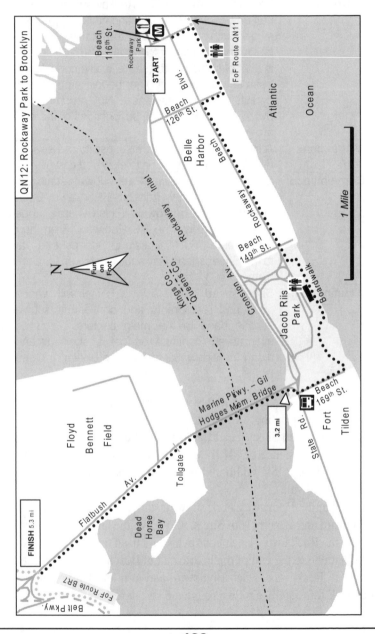

Here you find a vehicle-free street heading north—this is the lower end of Beach 169th Street. Follow this street north, past the barrier where it opens to traffic, and continue to the main road where there is a bus terminus. Cross the road here and bear right to join the pedestrian path onto the Gil Hodges Memorial Bridge (the only path is on the western side of the bridge).

Cross the bridge and follow the path past the tollgates. Shortly after this you face a choice. There is a light-controlled pedestrian crossing across Flatbush Avenue. If you cross here you can use a paved multiuse trail for the next mile. Alternatively, continue straight ahead on the concrete sidewalk, cutting out two road crossings but suffering a little poorer underfoot conditions and closer vehicular traffic. Make your own decision here.

Continue to the trail crossing light before the Belt Parkway. The trail here is that featured in route BR7 (Canarsie to Sheepshead Bay). We recommend you go to the left on this trail to get to Sheepshead Bay with its restaurants, bars, and subway station. It is 3.1 miles from the intersection to the center of Sheepshead Bay, on a mostly paved trail.

Other Routes

Cross Bay Boulevard connects the Howard Beach area to Broad Channel and Rockaway Beach, a distance of roughly five miles, with a pedestrian path all the way. There are always vehicles nearby but also plenty of fresh air. There are some excellent stretches with no motor vehicle intersections. There are some very ordinary stretches too.

Highland Park is located southwest of Forest Park on the Brook-lyn-Queens line. It is built around the decommissioned and drained Ridgewood Reservoir. It is primarily a nature preserve but you can run a loop around it (a little less than a mile). You can get to Highland Park on foot from the west end of Forest Park via the streets.

Running Clubs

Alley Pond Striders (www.apstriders.org)
A running/walking group for all ages and sexes, based at the Alley Pond park house on Winchester Boulevard north of Union Turnpike. The group exists to promote health, wellness, and plain old fun. There are

daily runs and walks. The group hosts an annual dinner dance, annual five-mile and 5K races, monthly walks, and refreshment days.
Email: gerardruiz@oasas.state.ny.us

College Point Road Runners Track Club (www.cprrtc.org)
The adult program is conducted year round with scheduled coached workouts and informal runs weekly. The club seeks committed, not necessarily super-fast, runners. There are group marathon training runs and post-run picnics April-October, plus other Marathon activities.
Email: cmcprrtc@aol.com

Forest Park Runners Club (forestparkrunners.org)
A club of runners and race walkers based in Forest Park, with members mostly in their 30s to 70s. It is an international group with over 20 countries represented. There are Saturday and Sunday morning and Wednesday evening group runs year-round. The club hosts the Forest Park Four-Mile Classic in May and a one-mile race series in summer.
Email: info@forestparkrunners.org

Hellgate Road Runners (hrr-online.org)
Located in Astoria, Queens, Hellgate was founded to promote fun and safety in competitive running. The club invites all comers to explore their web site and join them for group runs. Hellgate meets four days per week for group runs at the track in Astoria Park.
Email: jared@hrr-online.org

Quantum Athletics Club and Store (www.quantumathletics.net)
A small group which runs every Tuesday night on the Greenway Trail or in Kissena Park. All levels are welcome.
Email: info@quantumathletics.net

Quantum Feet Road Runners Club (www.qfrrc.org)
QFRRC strives to provide support for the athletic goals of each member, regardless of age, sex, competitive or fitness levels. QFRRC welcomes the indoor treadmill runner, amateur road racer and world-class distance runner alike. The club has group runs and sponsors at least one road race per year. Activities include monthly meetings, the Ocean to Sound Relay, Blue Line Run (two weeks prior to the New York City marathon), and social functions.
Email: info@qfrrc.org

5

The Bronx

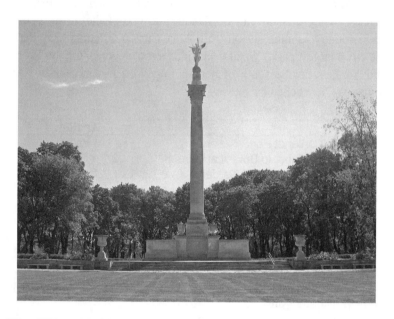

New York's northern-most borough, the Bronx, is home to roughly 1.4 million people and has an area of 42 square miles. This land was first settled by Europeans in 1639 when Jonas Bronck established a farm here. The land later became part of Westchester County in New York State. In the late 19th century, the various communities that now form the Bronx became part of New York City.[1]

The Bronx has some excellent parks that are ideal for on-foot exercise. There are several well maintained trails and places with abundant wildlife.

---

1   Chapter head photo: The Bronx Victory Memorial Column.

The borough overall does not have a shining reputation in terms of poverty and crime, but the situation has improved enormously since the 1970s, and most parts are now as safe as the rest of the city. Nevertheless, there are parts of the borough where caution is warranted. In particular, in the South Bronx, south of Fordham Road and west of the Bronx River, visitors might want to consult with locals before venturing out alone for on-foot exercise.

We have selected seven internal Bronx on-foot routes which, in our judgment, contain all the qualities of pleasant, interesting exercise venues. They include Van Cortlandt Park, one of the most popular cross-country running sites in New York City, and Pelham Bay Park, the city's largest park. We also included a route connecting the Bronx and Yonkers, in the south of neighboring Westchester County. All routes can be reached by subway.

Route	Distance
BX1 Van Cortlandt Park	Various
BX2 Van Cortlandt to Botanical Garden	2.1 miles one way
BX3 New York Botanical Garden	1.8 miles loop
BX4 Bronx River-Mosholu Parkways Loop	5.5 miles loop
BX5 Jerome Park Reservoir	2.0 miles loop
BX6 Botanical Garden to Pelham Bay	3.6 miles one way
BX7 Pelham Bay Park	5.7 miles loop
BX8 Van Cortlandt to Yonkers	5.0 miles one way

These routes can be linked to each other to form longer routes. Some possibilities are:

- Starting in Van Cortlandt Park, follow routes BX2 (Van Cortlandt to Botanical Garden) and BX6 (Botanical Garden to Pelham Bay) to end at the Pelham Bay Park subway station; total distance 5.7 miles;

- Starting in Van Cortland Park, follow route BX2 (Van Cortlandt to Botanical Garden), do a loop of the Botanical Garden following route BX3 (New York Botanical Garden), and return to Van Cortlandt Park; total distance 6.2 miles.

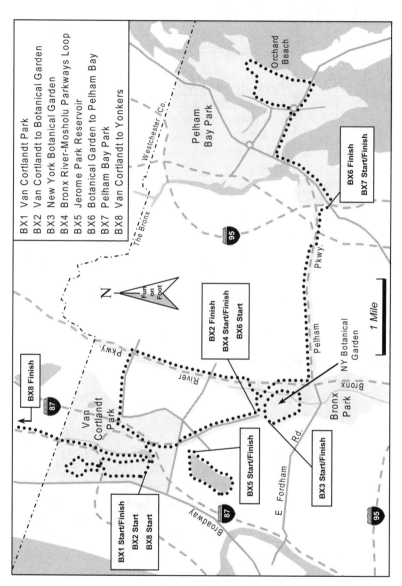

BX1 Van Cortlandt Park
BX2 Van Cortlandt to Botanical Garden
BX3 New York Botanical Garden
BX4 Bronx River-Mosholu Parkways Loop
BX5 Jerome Park Reservoir
BX6 Botanical Garden to Pelham Bay
BX7 Pelham Bay Park
BX8 Van Cortlandt to Yonkers

Orchard Beach

Pelham Bay Park

BX6 Finish
BX7 Start/Finish

Westchester Co.

The Bronx

95

N

Fun on Foot

Pelham Pkwy.

BX2 Finish
BX4 Start/Finish
BX6 Start

River Pkwy.

1 Mile

NY Botanical Garden

Bronx Park

BX8 Finish

87

Van Cortlandt Park

E Fordham Rd.

BX5 Start/Finish

BX3 Start/Finish

95

Broadway

87

BX1 Start/Finish
BX2 Start
BX8 Start

Bronx Routes

Van Cortlandt Park

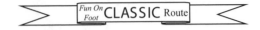

Distance	Various (Route BX1)
Comfort	Some very popular trails, with a range of conditions from paved circuits around fields to challenging grades through woods. Expect plenty of other on-foot exercisers around. Not suitable for inline skating.
Attractions	Woodlands with considerable wildlife. Excellent escape from the city's crowds and automobiles.
Convenience	Start and finish near the Van Cortlandt Park subway station at the end of the 1-train line. There is also parking nearby.
Destination	After your workout, there are some pleasant places to relax around Van Cortlandt Lake, and you can get a snack and soda or beer at the golf house. Alternatively, there are food and beverage places on Broadway near the subway.

Van Cortlandt Park, with 1,146 acres, can be easily reached by subway or car and has a number of attractions. Foremost, it has a substantial area of wilderness with leafy forests and considerable wildlife. The park was acquired by the city and designated as parkland in 1888.

There are many trails but their layout is complicated by four major impediments to east-west traversal of the park—the Henry Hudson Parkway, the Mosholu Parkway, the Major Deegan Expressway (Interstate 87), and a long, thin north-south-oriented golf course. Until you know the park well, you will appreciate having a trail map, which is available at the park's Nature Center. Even with the map, navigating the park can be challenging. Note that the condition of the different trails can vary enormously, from immaculate and wide to overgrown and barely passable.

The west side of the park is the best part for on-foot exercise. There are two particularly popular running/jogging/walking loops, and we feature both in this chapter:

- The 1.4-mile loop around the Parade Ground; and

- The network of trails known as the cross-country course, which connects to the Parade Ground and is used for cross-country races of varying lengths. We describe a 3.0-mile loop which generally tracks the frequently used 5K race course.

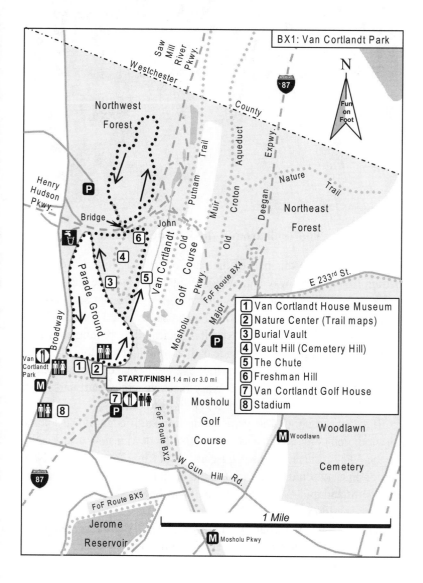

BX1: Van Cortlandt Park

1 Van Cortlandt House Museum
2 Nature Center (Trail maps)
3 Burial Vault
4 Vault Hill (Cemetery Hill)
5 The Chute
6 Freshman Hill
7 Van Cortlandt Golf House
8 Stadium

START/FINISH 1.4 mi or 3.0 mi

1 Mile

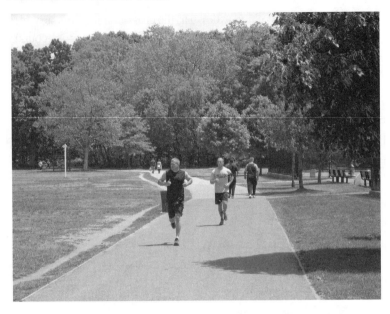

The Trail around the Parade Ground

You can get to this part of the park by subway to the end of the 1-train line at Broadway and W 242nd Street. Enter the park and go north a short distance to the southwest corner of the Parade Ground. Established in 1901, this open field was used by the National Guard until the end of World War I. Today it is dedicated to sporting activities, including running. There is a wide path around it, paved for part of the way and gravel for the rest. On-foot exercisers make their own earth tracks along the edge. Cross-country races generally start and finish somewhere on this field, known as *The Flats* to runners.

If you head about 150 yards along the south edge of the Parade Ground, you come to the historic Van Cortlandt Mansion, now known as the Van Cortlandt House Museum. Built in 1748, this was New York's first museum. Next to it is the Nature Center where there are restrooms and trail maps. We nominally declare this the start and finish point of our loops.

The 1.4-mile loop around the Parade Ground is flat and very popular, and needs no further discussion. The 3.0-mile loop is more challenging and interesting.

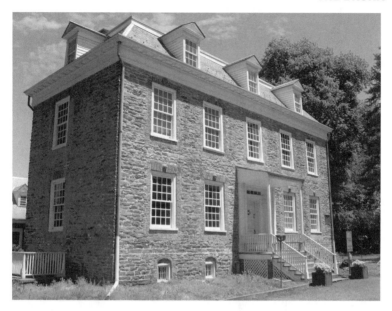

The Van Cortlandt House Museum

Proceed counterclockwise around the Parade Ground to the trail bearing off to the right with the characteristic tortoise-and-hare sign used to designate the cross-country course. Follow this part of the course, known as *The Chute*, through the woods up the edge of the golf course. You pass a trail heading off perpendicularly to the left. This leads to ruins of what used to be the Van Cortlandt family burial vault, and also gives access to more challenging variations of the cross-country course that negotiate Vault Hill.

Continuing up The Chute, as you approach the Henry Hudson Parkway, the trail swings left and climbs upward. This section is known as *Freshman Hill*. It leads you up to a four-way trail intersection. Take the path to the right, across the footbridge over Henry Hudson Parkway into the Northwest Forest section of the park.

There are many trails twisting and turning through the Northwest Forest and, to avoid the risk of becoming lost, we recommend sticking to the well maintained, tortoise-and-hare marked cross-country course. Turn right after the bridge and follow the twisting course 1.3 miles, first northward and then back to the bridge across Henry Hudson Parkway. This section is known as the *Back Hills* part of the course.

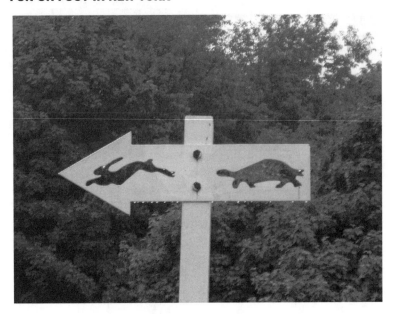

The Cross-Country Course Icon

VARIATION

Vault Hill, also known as Cemetery Hill, is a challenging, steep part of the cross-country trail network that you can add in when running The Chute. You can get to it either from the perpendicular trail near the vault or from another trail junction further along The Chute, near the start of Freshman Hill. Follow the tortoise-and-hare signs first south and then around a hairpin bend, taking you just east of the vault. Continue up and then down Vault Hill to emerge at the four-way trail intersection.

Cross the bridge back to the four-way trail intersection. Vault Hill is straight ahead. For our featured route, go right and follow the trail around to the northern end of the Parade Ground. Pick up the loop trail counterclockwise around the Parade Ground and back to the start point. Continue repeating as many 1.4-mile and/or 3.0-mile circuits as you wish.

When done, there are a couple of choices of place to wind down. The closest is the Van Cortlandt golf house where you can get a snack and a soda or beer. From the southeast corner of the Parade Ground, follow the paved trail down to the edge of Van Cortlandt Lake and around the bottom end of the lake to the clubhouse of the nation's oldest public golf course (established 1895). Alternatively, head back to the Van Cortlandt Park subway station on Broadway. Across Broadway there are some food and beverage joints should you need them. If you are mainly thirsty, try Dorney and Malone's Irish watering hole.

* * * *

Van Cortlandt Park has several other trails of interest to runners, joggers, and walkers, most notably:

- The 400-meter artificial surface running track in the stadium at the southwest corner of the park;
- The Old Putnam Trail, a rail trail starting at the lower end of Van Cortlandt Lake across from the golf clubhouse and extending northward into Westchester County; see our route BX8 (Van Cortlandt to Yonkers) for more details on this and the following trail;
- The Old Croton Aqueduct Trail, which also extends northward into Westchester County;
- The John Muir Nature Trail takes you from the Northwest Forest pedestrian bridge to the east side of the park to connect with the Old Croton Aqueduct Trail and the woods in the northeast part of the park.

However, in our experience, the last two trails are not well maintained and we suggest you only attempt them if you have company and limited expectations.

Van Cortlandt to Botanical Garden

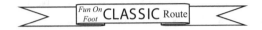

Distance	2.1 miles one way (Route BX2)
Comfort	Excellent underfoot conditions on paved pedestrian/bicycle paths, partly through the park and partly in a pleasant residential neighborhood. Expect plenty of on-foot exercisers and cyclists around. Mostly good for inline skating but there are some serious uphill grades.
Attractions	This is a very pleasant route with the appeal of connecting two places that are of great interest to on-foot exercisers.
Convenience	Start near the Van Cortlandt Park subway station at the end of the 1-train line. Finish near the entrance to the New York Botanical Garden and the Metro North Botanical Garden station. There are subway stations less than a mile away from the finish.
Destination	The New York Botanical Garden has some outstanding botanical displays, food outlets, and trails for on-foot exercisers. See route BX3 (New York Botanical Garden) for more details. If reversing this route, the destination is Van Cortlandt Park with further on-foot trails, food and beverage outlets, and a convenient subway station.

There is a beautiful trail from Van Cortlandt Park down to the New York Botanical Garden, following the Mosholu Parkway. You can use this route in various ways, including connecting between the Bronx's two big parks—Van Cortlandt and Pelham Bay. Or maybe you just want to plan a day seeing both Van Cortlandt Park and the Botanical Garden.

We start at the same place as our previous route, by the Van Cortlandt House Museum on the edge of the Parade Ground in Van Cortlandt Park. From the southeast corner of the Parade Ground, follow the paved trail down to the edge of Van Cortlandt Lake and around the bottom end of the lake to the Van Cortlandt golf house.

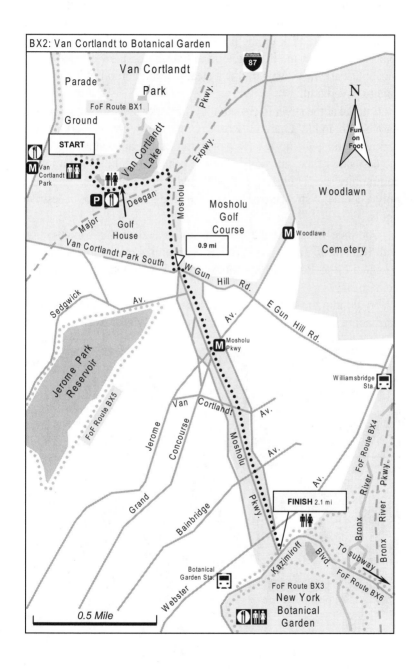

BX2: Van Cortlandt to Botanical Garden

Van Cortlandt
Parade
Park
FoF Route BX1
Ground

START

Van Cortlandt
Park

Van Cortlandt Lake

Deegan

Major

Golf House

Van Cortlandt Park South

Sedgwick

Av.

Jerome Park Reservoir

FoF Route BX5

Mosholu

Mosholu Golf Course

0.9 mi

W Gun Hill Rd.

E Gun Hill Rd.

Av.

Mosholu Pkwy

Av.

Van Cortlandt

Av.

Av.

Jerome

Concourse

Grand

Bainbridge

Mosholu Pkwy.

Kazimiroff

Webster

Botanical Garden Sta.

FINISH 2.1 mi

FoF Route BX3
New York Botanical Garden

Woodlawn

Woodlawn

Cemetery

Williamsbridge Sta.

FoF Route BX4

Bronx River Pkwy.

To subway

Bronx River

FoF Route BX6

Blvd.

N
Fun on Foot

0.5 Mile

From the golf house, go north on the beautiful trail along the lake's east edge. This is a popular place for school children excursions, near the nature trails. Pick up the paved bike path and follow it under the road ramp and around in a big loop to track along the west side of the Mosholu Parkway. This trail is a steady uphill climb but it is a good quality paved trail.

Emerge at the street intersection of the parkway with Van Cortlandt Park South and W Gun Hill Road. Cross the east-west road and the parkway and pick up a new paved multiuse trail continuing down the east side of the parkway. This is a beautiful trail through a lovely community area. In spring enjoy the many flowering trees. There are only a couple of street crossings and they are quiet and have pedestrian lights.

Continue following the parkway to its end at the T-intersection with Kazimiroff Boulevard. This is the nominal end of this route. To continue on to Pelham Bay, follow route BX6 (Botanical Garden to Pelham Bay).

To get into the Botanical Garden go right along Kazimiroff Boulevard about 200 yards, near the entrance to the Metro North Botanical

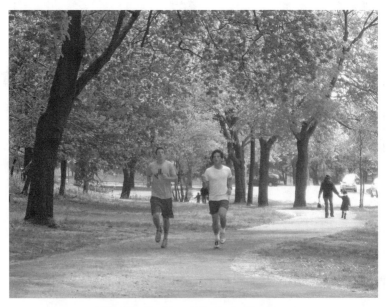

The Trail along Mosholu Parkway

Garden station. Cross Kazimiroff Boulevard at the pedestrian crossing and enter the Botanical Garden here. For more details, see route BX3 (New York Botanical Garden).

VARIATION

To continue on-foot to the nearest subway station (0.8 mile extra), turn left on the trail along Kazimiroff Boulevard. You pass a seasonal restroom at a playground at the trail junction with the Bronx River Greenway. Continue following the road and cross the Bronx River. Continue to the intersection with Allerton Avenue. Proceed east three blocks on Allerton Avenue to the 2-train station.

New York Botanical Garden

Distance	1.8 miles loop (Route BX3)
Comfort	Excellent underfoot conditions on paved vehicle-free roads. Expect to share the roads with plenty of wandering plant lovers plus some other on-foot exercisers, but the roads are wide and there is usually plenty of room for everyone. Inline skating is prohibited.
Attractions	This is a beautiful loop through areas of attractive and sometimes stunning foliage.
Convenience	Start and end at the garden entrance on Kazimiroff Boulevard, across the street from the Metro North Botanical Garden station. This is 0.1 mile from terminal points of routes BX2 (Van Cortlandt to Botanical Garden), BX4 (Bronx River-Mosholu Parkways Loop), and BX6 (Botanical Garden to Pelham Bay), so consider tacking this route onto one of those. The Allerton subway station is less than a mile away. If driving, the main parking lot is on the west edge of the garden, near the visitor center entrance.
Destination	The New York Botanical Garden has some outstanding botanical displays, food outlets, and access to public transit and other on-foot trails.

The New York Botanical Garden is one of the most renowned gardens in the nation. It also has many wide, spacious trails through it, well suited to outdoor exercise. Furthermore, while there is a charge for some of the exhibits, there is no charge for general admission to the garden or for use of the trails. One caution: the garden is closed on Mondays, except for federal holidays.

We start at the entrance to the gardens across Kazimiroff Boulevard from the Metro North Botanical Garden station. This is 0.1 mile from the termination point of our other routes noted in the table. We believe that, from an exercise perspective, you will most likely appreciate this route if you tack it onto one of those longer routes.

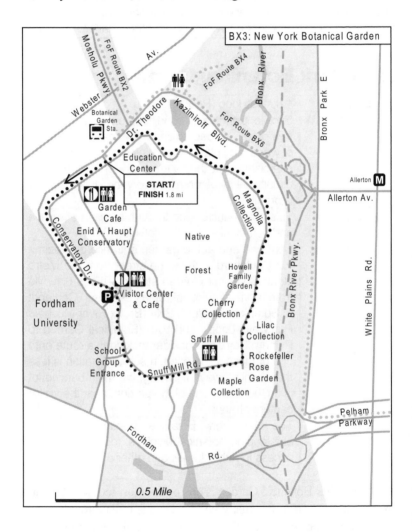

Inside the garden's entrance is a ticket and information kiosk. You can pick up a trail map here or at the visitor center by the main entrance.

The route we suggest is the main paved loop around the garden. Depending on season, you may be dazzled by the beauty of the cherry, lilac, and magnolia collections along this loop. Head south on the paved road past the Garden Café and swing left around to the main entrance and visitor center. Continue straight ahead to the school group entrance and head north on Snuff Mill Road, following the signs to Snuff Mill and the Rockefeller Rose Garden. Keep heading counterclockwise on the main road, past the Howell Family Garden and the Magnolia Collection, to arrive eventually at the education center. Go through the car park and back to your start point.

There are many other route choices and we encourage you to explore. However, you face a risk of meeting congestion on the narrower trails.

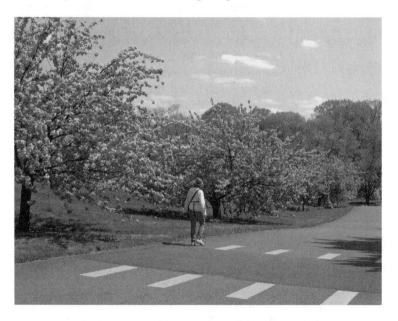

Flowering Cherry Trees in the Botanical Garden

Bronx River-Mosholu Parkways Loop

Distance	5.5 miles loop (Route BX4)
Comfort	3.3 miles are on good paved multiuse trails along the two parkways; 1.2 miles are on a less well maintained paved trail in Van Cortlandt Park; and one mile is on the sidewalk of a lightly-to-moderately trafficked street with minimal cross-traffic encounters. Expect some other people around, except on the Van Cortlandt Park stretch which is little used. (You might want to avoid doing this part without company.) Inline skating is good in parts but not recommended overall owing to some substantial grades and a large staircase to negotiate.
Attractions	This is a very pleasant route with few cross-traffic incursions and a shady environment. A good workout for a runner in training.
Convenience	Start and end anywhere on the loop, including Van Cortlandt Park, the Botanical Garden, or any of several subway stations (see map). We nominally start and finish near the entrance to the Botanical Garden and the Metro North Botanical Garden station. This is the end point of route BX2 (Van Cortlandt to Botanical Garden) and start point of route BX6 (Botanical Garden to Pelham Bay).
Destination	You can choose to finish at the Botanical Garden or Van Cortlandt Park, or add on route BX6 (Botanical Garden to Pelham Bay) to end at Pelham Bay Park.

The Bronx has two very pleasant parkway trails that are maintained by the city. The first, known as the Mosholu Parkway Greenway, extends from the south edge of Van Cortlandt Park down past the Botanical Garden to Bronx Park East. We used that in route BX2 (Van Cortlandt to Botanical Garden). The second, known as the Bronx River Greenway, extends north from near the Botanical Garden up the Bronx River valley to E 233rd Street. (There are plans to extend the latter north into Westchester County, but at publication time the part north of E 233rd Street is not sufficiently developed to recommend it.)

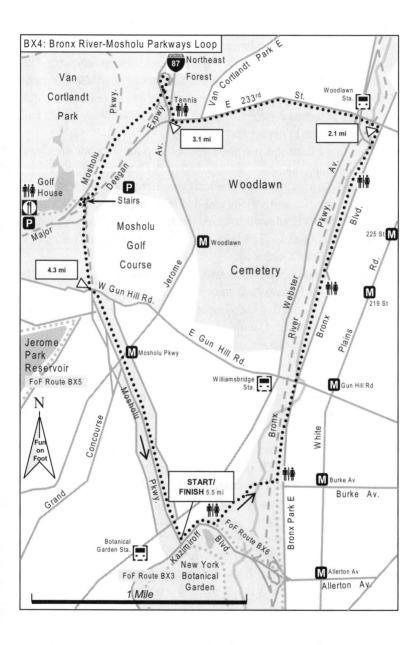

BX4: Bronx River-Mosholu Parkways Loop

Van Cortlandt Park

Northeast Forest

87

Tennis

Van Cortlandt Park E

E 233rd St.

Woodlawn Sta.

3.1 mi

2.1 mi

Golf House

Stairs

P

P

Woodlawn

Mosholu Golf Course

M Woodlawn

Cemetery

225 St M

219 St M

4.3 mi

W Gun Hill Rd.

Jerome

Webster

Bronx

River

Plains Rd.

Jerome Park Reservoir

FoF Route BX5

M Mosholu Pkwy

E Gun Hill Rd.

Williamsbridge Sta.

M Gun Hill Rd

N

Fun on Foot

Concourse

Mosholu

White

M Burke Av

Burke Av.

Grand

START/ FINISH 5.5 mi

Pkwy.

Bronx Park E

Botanical Garden Sta.

Kazimiroff Blvd.

FoF Route BX6

M Allerton Av

Allerton Av.

FoF Route BX3

New York Botanical Garden

1 Mile

What is particularly interesting to the on-footer is that we can build a four-segment loop that uses those two greenway trails as two of the segments. The third segment is the sidewalk of E 233rd Street along the northern edge of Woodlawn Cemetery—apart from being a quite challenging uphill workout, this is a nice, friendly loop segment. The fourth segment is a paved trail through the eastern side of Van Cortlandt Park. It is mostly a good trail but has a couple of less-than-ideal parts, including a sometimes-overgrown path through dark, lonely woods and a long set of stairs to negotiate.

Overall, we think this is a good on-foot loop for someone seeking a more challenging outing.

We chose to start near the Botanical Garden entrance where Mosholu Parkway meets Kazimiroff Boulevard. Head east on the multiuse trail along Kazimiroff Boulevard towards the Bronx River. You come to a major trail junction. Go left here, past the playground and restrooms, up the Bronx River Greenway.

The trail leads over a bridge across the Bronx River and then under the Bronx River Parkway. It then joins the trail along the east edge of Bronx Park—go left at the T-junction. This is a very pleasant trail, mostly through parkland, with one short section on a street sidewalk. There are restrooms along the way.

As you approach the E 233rd Street intersection, cross the parkway ramp and continue to the intersection. Turn left, go over the parkway, and proceed up E 233rd Street. This section of the route involves quite a long climb. Just before Jerome Avenue, you come to a set of tennis courts on your right, with restrooms adjacent.

Go right at the Jerome Avenue light and then cross the street where you see a little path on the other side. Follow this path along the edge of the highway ramp and over the Major Deegan Expressway. The path then curls right and runs along the side of the expressway under the ramp overpass. Shortly after, it peels off to the right and into the woods. The path is paved, so is easy to follow even though it is not maintained well and may be somewhat overgrown. The Old Croton Aqueduct trail joins this paved trail along this stretch but it is sometimes so overgrown you will not notice it. This is why we chose not to cover this part of the Aqueduct trail.

The paved trail emerges on the eastern edge of Mosholu Parkway and follows that road a short distance. It then drifts back to track the

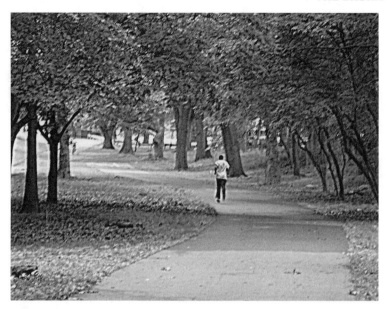

The Bronx River Greenway

expressway and crosses the parkway. At this point you come to a set of steps leading down to the level of the parkway roadway. Go down to join the paved multiuse trail that links the Van Cortland golf house to W Gun Hill Road. Follow the trail south along the parkway.

VARIATION

You can end your route in Van Cortlandt Park by taking the trail to the left, passing by the lake to the golf house and beyond. You eventually come to facilities and the Van Cortlandt Park 1-train subway station.

Emerge at the street intersection of the parkway with Van Cortlandt Park South and W Gun Hill Road. Cross the east-west road and the parkway and pick up a new paved multiuse trail continuing down the east side of the parkway. Follow the parkway to its end at the T-intersection with Kazimiroff Boulevard.

Jerome Park Reservoir

Distance	2.0 miles loop (Route BX5)
Comfort	Excellent underfoot conditions on quiet street sidewalks or paved pedestrian paths. Expect plenty of on-foot exercisers around. Not recommended for inline skating.
Attractions	This is a very pleasant route with no traffic incursions and a generally quiet, shady environment.
Convenience	Start near the intersection of Sedgwick Avenue and Mosholu Parkway, off route BX2 (Van Cortlandt to Botanical Garden), a short trek from Van Cortlandt Park, and near the Mosholu Parkway subway station. Consider combining with route BX4 (Bronx River-Mosholu Parkways Loop).
Destination	No compelling destination, but consider linking this route with our other nearby Bronx routes.

Jerome Park was a racecourse in the latter part of the nineteenth century, until it was acquired and converted to a reservoir as part of the New Croton Aqueduct system. It still serves as part of New York City's water supply system today.

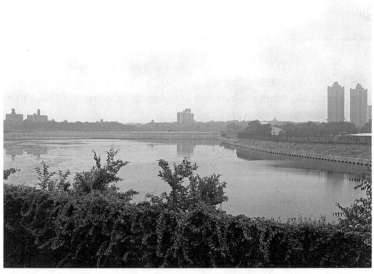

Jerome Park Reservoir

The reservoir has a long history as a place for on-foot exercise, although its appeal has been muted for many years by the presence of a large protective fence, keeping people well away from the water. Today it is still a popular place for locals to exercise, providing a two-mile circuit devoid of vehicle interruptions. Its proximity to several educational institutions helps keep it popular.

You can get here easily by subway or on-foot from Van Cortlandt Park via the streets or route BX2 (Van Cortlandt to Botanical Garden).

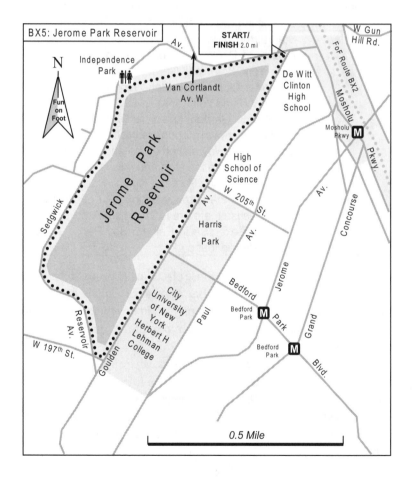

Botanical Garden to Pelham Bay

Distance	3.6 miles one way (Route BX6)
Comfort	Good underfoot conditions on paved pedestrian/ bicycle paths, mostly through a pleasant residential neighborhood. There are moderately busy roads nearby throughout the route and there are several street crossings. Expect plenty of on-foot exercisers around. OK for inline skating.
Attractions	This is a pleasant route with the appeal of connecting two great on-foot exercise venues.
Convenience	Start at the intersection of Mosholu Parkway and Kazimiroff Boulevard, near the entrance to the New York Botanical Garden and the Botanical Garden station on the Metro North Harlem Line. This is the end point of route BX2 (Van Cortlandt to Botanical Garden) and route BX4 (Bronx River-Mosholu Parkways Loop). Finish at the Pelham Bay Park subway station at the end of the 6-train line. This is also the start and finish point of route BX7 (Pelham Bay Park).
Destination	Either make the subway station your destination, in which case there are food joints nearby, or plan for further exercise in Pelham Bay Park. There are facilities in that park.

While the most exciting on-foot exercise places in the Bronx are the Van Cortlandt Park vicinity and Pelham Bay Park, a particularly interesting route is the connection between those places. In this route description, we cover that connection—yet another beautifully maintained and comfortable Bronx trail.

We start near the Botanical Garden entrance where Mosholu Parkway meets Kazimiroff Boulevard. This allows you to easily add this route onto route BX2 (Van Cortlandt to Botanical Garden). Head east on the multiuse trail along Kazimiroff Boulevard towards the Bronx River. You come to a major trail junction. Continue straight ahead following the road here.

Cross the Bronx River and continue to the street intersection at Allerton Avenue and Bronx Park E. Go to the right, crossing the street at the pedestrian crossing, and pick up the trail through the park down to Pelham Parkway.

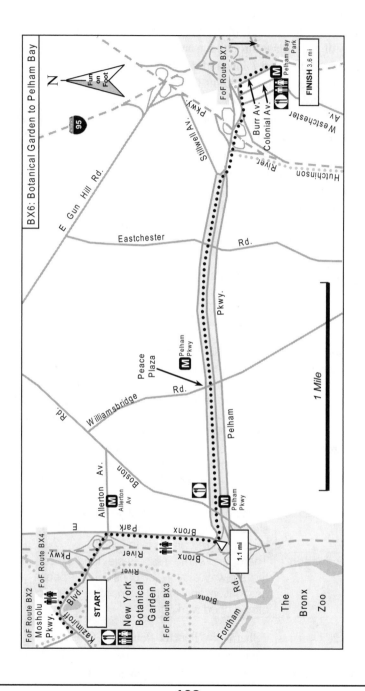

BX6: Botanical Garden to Pelham Bay

At Pelham Parkway, go immediately left on the multiuse trail. This is a lovely trail through immaculate residential communities. Expect plenty of pedestrians throughout, and relatively few cyclists. At Boston Road there are food joints and a subway station. At Williamsbridge Road pass Peace Plaza, with its Gulf War memorial.

At Stillwell Avenue cross the parkway at the traffic light and continue east. Go over the rail tracks and the Hutchinson River Parkway. There are a couple of tricky ramps here—be very careful that no vehicles are coming before crossing.

After the Hutchinson River Parkway you can choose to either go straight ahead to Pelham Bay Park or bear right on Colonial Avenue or Burr Avenue to the local commercial area and the subway station. There are some reasonable food joints here if you need nourishment and there are restrooms in the subway station.

Pelham Bay Park

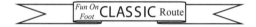

Distance	5.7 miles loop (Route BX7)
Comfort	Good-to-excellent underfoot conditions with plenty of on-foot exercisers and cyclists around. Most of the route is on paved pedestrian/bicycle paths, with a short section on an unpaved walking path. Mostly OK for inline skating.
Attractions	Plenty of fresh air and escape from heavy automobile traffic. Some beautiful views of Long Island Sound and the relaxation of passing by a long sandy beach.
Convenience	Start and finish at the Pelham Bay Park subway station at the northern end of the 6-train line. There is also ample parking in the park.
Destination	There are some reasonable food places near the subway station, or consider the beach your destination and spend some time relaxing there after a good workout.

With 2,764 acres, Pelham Bay Park is New York City's largest park. There is great running or walking here for Bronx residents. It can also be reached from Manhattan and other locations via subway.

The park can be considered to comprise three main segments. The Pelham South segment, near the subway station, contains sporting fields, playgrounds, and other facilities. It includes a 440-yard running track in the recreational complex. The northwest segment comprises two golf courses, a riding stable, bridle trail, marshlands, and woods. The eastern segment comprises mainly Orchard Beach and surrounding facilities, plus the Hunter Island nature preservation area.

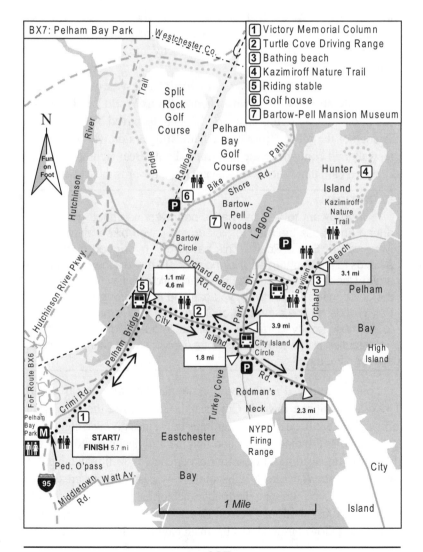

Pelham Bay Park has various trails of differing quality. The most dependable trails are the well-maintained paved bike paths. Many of the other trails marked on the park map are of questionable quality and sometimes impassable. We therefore constructed a route that mostly uses those paved paths. We elected to build a loop starting and ending at the subway station and extending to Orchard Beach. There are many ways to vary this loop to satisfy your own tastes.

Take a subway 6 train to its northern terminus, the Pelham Bay Park station. The trip can take a long time from Manhattan if you are on a local train, so try to catch an express. From the station there is a pedestrian overpass over Interstate 95 directly into the park. There are restrooms here.

Bear left, generally tracking Crimi Road. Go past the majestic Bronx Victory Memorial Column, which honors Bronx World War I veterans. (See photo at head of this chapter.) Pick up the paved bike path along the edge of the road. Cross the Pelham Bridge (a drawbridge) on the sidewalk and continue to the first traffic light. Bear right and pick up the paved path that follows City Island Road towards the east.

VARIATION

If you want to visit the park's northwest segment, go straight ahead and cross the road to pick up the paved bike trail along the west side of Shore Road. This paved trail is of good quality and extends to the northern edge of the park. To make a loop you can go around the Split Rock Golf Course on the bridle trail, which starts near the golf house. Alternatively, you can find trails through the Bartow-Pell Woods on the east side of Shore Road. We have, however, found these unpaved trails of questionable quality, often overgrown. An attraction is that you can stop for a drink or snack on the way back at the golf house.

Follow the paved eastbound trail around the traffic circle at Park Drive and continue towards City Island. Just before the City Island bridge there are breaks in the guardrails both sides giving a convenient place to cross the road. Cross and find the trail heading into the trees. This is an unpaved trail but, in our experience, is well maintained. It takes you to the water, with sights of the City Island marina area across the water. Keep following the trail to the north. It brings you out in a grassy field just south of Orchard Beach. Go up to the beach promenade and follow it around past the main pavilion. There are restrooms and outlets for snacks, beer, and sodas here. Orchard Beach is a very pleasant bathing beach, so you might choose to take a dip while here.

To complete our loop, go around the pavilion and behind it, skirting the enormous car park, to pick up the paved multiuse trail heading south and west.

VARIATION

If you continue along the beach north of the Orchard Beach Pavilion, you come to the trailhead of the Kazimiroff Nature Trail. This is a pleasant nature trail but not really amenable to serious on-foot exercise.

Follow the paved trail along Park Drive, past the first major road intersection to the pedestrian crossing before the traffic circle at City Island Road. Cross the pedestrian crossing and take the paved trail here back along City Island Road on its north side. Pass the Turtle Cove driving range and mini-golf center. There are public restrooms here and you can buy snacks, beer, and sodas.

Continue back to the traffic light. Cross City Island Road and head back south towards Pelham Bridge. Retrace your steps to the subway station.

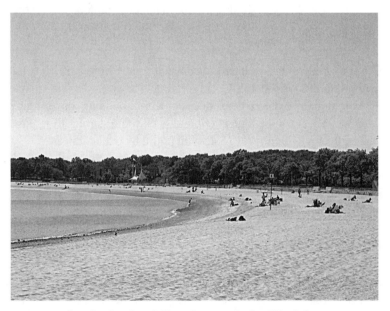

Sandy Orchard Beach on a Quiet Weekday

Van Cortlandt to Yonkers

Distance	5.0 miles one way (Route BX8)
Comfort	The first 1.5 miles are on a wide, unpaved, shady park trail. The next 1.8 miles are on a well-maintained paved multiuse rail trail. The final 1.7 miles are on a mix of street sidewalks and a less well maintained unpaved trail behind residences. Expect to pass other on-foot exercisers and cyclists in the first 3.5 miles, with fewer on the final 1.7 miles. Not suitable for inline skating, except on the paved rail trail section.
Attractions	This route offers excellent running conditions. There is abundant wildlife on the first section.
Convenience	Start near the Van Cortlandt Park subway station at the end of the 1-train line. Finish at the Yonkers station on the Metro North Hudson Line.
Destination	Yonkers Center has food and beverage establishments and a Metro North rail station. You can also choose to continue further north along the Old Croton Aqueduct Trail; see Chapter 8 for details. If reversing this route, the destination is Van Cortlandt Park with further on-foot trails, food and beverage outlets, and a convenient subway station.

Our final route in this chapter is a connector route from our Bronx trail network to the Westchester County trail network described in Chapter 8. You might use this route as one segment in building longer routes. Alternatively, it can be a great out-and-back route starting from either end, or treat it as a one-way route with return by public transit.

We start near the Botanical Garden entrance where Mosholu Parkway meets Kazimiroff Boulevard. This allows you to easily add this route onto route BX2 (Van Cortlandt to Botanical Garden). Head east on the multiuse trail along Kazimiroff Boulevard towards the Bronx River. You come to a major trail junction. Continue straight ahead following the road here.

There are two trails from Van Cortlandt Park heading north across the city boundary into Westchester County—the Old Putnam Trail and the Old Croton Aqueduct Trail. Since the former is well maintained and well used and the latter tends to be unkempt and lonely, we chose

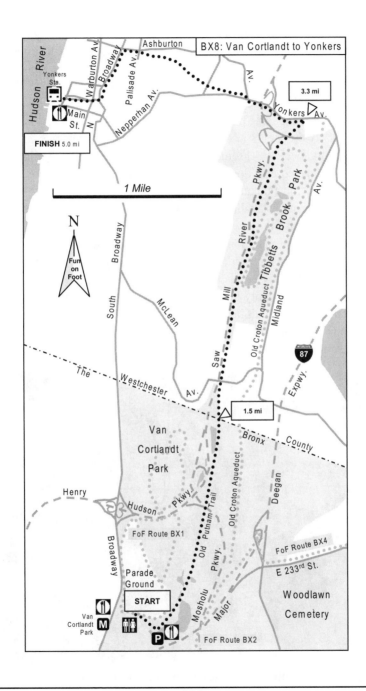

BX8: Van Cortlandt to Yonkers

to cover only the former. From where the Old Putnam Trail intersects Yonkers Avenue in Yonkers, you can conveniently connect with the extension of the Old Croton Aqueduct Trail to either get to Yonkers Center and the Metro North railroad station or follow the Aqueduct further north in Westchester County. For the latter, see route WC1 (Yonkers to Dobbs Ferry).

We start at the same place as our previous Van Cortland Park routes, by the Van Cortlandt House Museum on the edge of the Parade Ground in Van Cortlandt Park. From the southeast corner of the Parade Ground, follow the paved trail down to the edge of Van Cortlandt Lake. You intersect the Old Putnam Trail just before reaching the lake. Go left along what is unmistakably the bed of an old railroad. The Old Putnam Railroad, which ran between High Bridge and Brewster, New York, ceased passenger operations in 1958 and was fully shut down in 1981.

The Van Cortlandt Park part of this trail is unpaved but excellent underfoot and shady. It also abounds with wildlife. When you reach the Westchester County line, conditions change. It becomes a nicely maintained paved, multiuse trail.

You are now in Yonkers. For runners, Yonkers is a significant place because it is home to the nation's second-oldest marathon, first run in

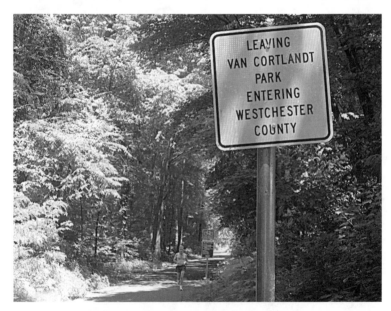

Conditions Change at the County Line

1907. The Yonkers Marathon and Half Marathon are held in September. The route is very hilly and challenging and consequently attracts only a small field.

The rail trail takes you along the west edge of Tibbetts Brook Park. This is a pleasant park and you can run loops here if you wish. There are access paths to the park from the trail at a few points.

Continue on the trail to the stairs down to the left, just before the old rail bridge over Yonkers Avenue. Go down the stairs to the sidewalk of Yonkers Avenue and follow it to the left. This takes you over the Saw Mill River Parkway. At the next light-controlled intersection, cross Yonkers Avenue and continue in the same direction on the other side.

After a short distance, a grassy pedestrian path peels off to the right. This is a segment of the Old Croton Aqueduct trail. (See Chapter 8 for further discussion of the Aqueduct trail.) This trail leads to Palisade Avenue, just south of Ashburton Avenue. While this is a convenient and historically interesting trail, when we were last there it had a significant problem—it was inundated with trash and seemed very poorly maintained. The Friends of the Old Croton Aqueduct, the very dedicated not-for-profit advocate group supporting the preservation of the Aqueduct, told me they are painfully aware of the poor state of the trail in Yonkers. They are actively working with the State Parks Office and local residents and community groups to correct the problem and they anticipate that these efforts will lead to greatly improved conditions soon. We look forward to that happening and encourage readers to bear with any less-than-ideal conditions in the meantime.

The trail emerges at Ashburton Avenue. Follow that street west to North Broadway. Here, you have a choice of either following the next section of the Aqueduct trail (see route WC1 in Chapter 8) or heading to Yonkers Center to catch a Metro North Hudson Line train. For the latter, turn left along North Broadway and proceed downhill to end in the vicinity of Main Street. The Yonkers Metro North station is at the west end of Main Street. Trains from here can take you to the Bronx or Manhattan. There is also a weekday, peak-hour ferry service to the World Financial Center from here. There are some reasonable eating and drinking establishments in Main Street, if you need a break before continuing your outing.

Other Routes

The **Hutchinson River Parkway Greenway** runs from Pelham Parkway, a little west of Pelham Bay Park, southward to the Interstate-95 corridor. It is an excellent-quality paved multiuse trail but unfortunately it does not lead anywhere very interesting. At the south end, the trail takes you over the parkway and under the interstate highway, to emerge at Bruckner Boulevard and Brush Avenue. You can follow Bruckner Boulevard across Westchester Creek, giving access to Clason Point and Sound View Park via the local streets. However, these streets are very ordinary, so we chose not to feature this route at present. There are plans to build more multiuse trails around Clason Point. If and when these are built and link up with the Hutchinson River Parkway Greenway, we may have a very appealing route here. One could go, for example, to Sound View Park and up the Bronx River Parkway corridor to the subway line at Westchester Avenue. Keep this one in mind for future years.

Running Clubs

Van Cortlandt Track Club (www.vctc.org)
Open to all runners, regardless of ability or experience. Some members have been running for many years, others just for a few months. Some regularly win awards at local races; others prefer not to race at all. Members share a love of running and the camaraderie that develops as they hit the roads and trails together. There are group runs Saturdays at 8:00 am and speed workouts Tuesdays at 7:00 pm. Hosted races include the Urban Environmental Challenge 10K trail race in April, the Riverdale Ramble 10K road race in June in the streets of Riverdale, and the Cross-Country Summer Series 5K, every other Thursday at 7:00 pm, late May through mid-August.
Email: Refer to website.

6

Staten Island

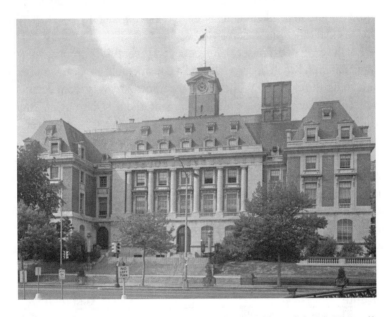

NewYork's southernmost borough occupies an island, 13.9 miles long and 7.3 miles wide. With a land area of 58.5 square miles and a population under a half-million, its population density is far lower than the other four boroughs. This borough has a charm of its own![1]

Staten Island is accessible by road from Brooklyn via the Verrazano-Narrows Bridge and from New Jersey via three bridges.

An equally important means of access is by the famous Staten Island Ferry, which operates between the lower tip of Manhattan and Staten Island's Saint George ferry terminal. It is a high capacity and very

---

1   Chapter head photo: Staten Island Borough Hall, © New York Public Library, reproduced with permission.

efficient ferry system and is free of charge. While it is of tremendous importance to many commuters, the Staten Island Ferry is also a major tourist attraction. It offers visitors a free tour of Upper New York Bay, passing close by the Statue of Liberty. The trip takes about 25 minutes one way.

Staten Island became part of New York City in 1898 but remained relatively undeveloped and remote from the other boroughs until the building of the Verrazano-Narrows Bridge in 1964. Even today, Staten Island has a somewhat different character to the other boroughs. It is largely suburban residential in nature and locals generally consider "the City" as that other place, across the water.

For the on-foot exerciser, there are several beautifully groomed parks, an outstanding beach boardwalk, and a considerable area of wilderness with trails through it. While these resources are very convenient to the local residents, they are less convenient to out-of-borough visitors, which may or may not add to their appeal to you. We shall, however, do our best to explain ways for everyone to get to the best trails.

As to public transit, there are no subways on Staten Island. Transit systems predominantly fan out from the Saint George ferry terminal and include the Staten Island Railway, a rapid transit system extending to the southern tip of the island, plus a comprehensive bus network. To a large extent, these ground transport systems are scheduled to link up with ferry departures and arrivals.

We chose to feature eight on-foot routes in this book.

Route	Distance
SI1 The Ferry to Fort Wadsworth	3.0 miles one way
SI2 South and Midland Beaches	3.3 miles one way
SI3 Miller Field	Various
SI4 Great Kills Park	4.2 miles out/back
SI5 Silver Lake Park	1.5 miles loop
SI6 Clove Lakes Park	Various
SI7 Staten Island Greenbelt	Various
SI8 Conference House Park	1.8 miles loop

Some of these routes can be linked together to form longer routes. Some possibilities are:

- Starting at the ferry terminal, do route SI1 (The Ferry to Fort Wadsworth), route SI2 (South and Midland Beaches), and

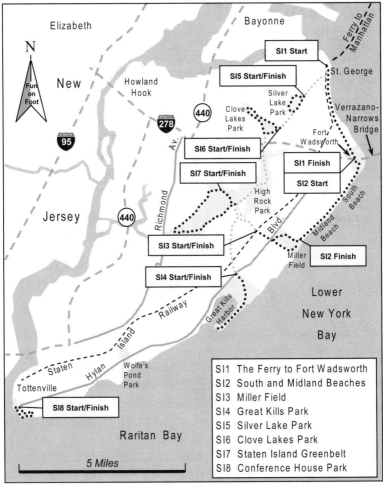

Staten Island Routes

route SI3 (Miller Field) to end at the New Dorp Staten Island Railway station and return to the ferry by train; total on-foot distance 7.9 miles one way;

• In the various route descriptions we have pointed out some connectors between routes, including connectors between: SI3 and SI7; SI4 and SI7; SI5 and SI6; and SI6 and SI7. You have many opportunities for linking up good on-foot routes on Staten Island to design longer outings of your own.

The Ferry to Fort Wadsworth

Distance	3.0 miles one way (Route SI1)
Comfort	This route is mostly on sidewalks of streets that are not heavily trafficked. Do not expect many other pedestrians. Not recommended for inline skating.
Attractions	The appeal of this route is it takes you on-foot from the ferry to one of Staten Island's most interesting and scenic destinations, historic Fort Wadsworth. Furthermore, from here you can quickly get on-foot to some outstanding on-foot environments along the island's top beaches.
Convenience	Start at the Saint George ferry terminal. Finish at the visitor center of Fort Wadsworth. The S51 bus connects the start and finish.
Destination	Fort Wadsworth, one of the nation's oldest military installations, has several historic points of interest and impressive views of New York Harbor.

We have included this route not for its beauty but for its practical value in connecting a visitor arriving by ferry to some of the most interesting and beautiful parts of the island. This route ends at Fort Wadsworth, itself a very interesting destination, nestled in the shadow of the majestic Verrazano-Narrows Bridge. The route also connects to route SI2 (South and Midland Beaches), which offers some outstanding running conditions and ocean beach scenery.

Start at the Saint George ferry terminal. Ferries to here from the lower end of Manhattan are frequent and free. For a city visitor staying in Manhattan, a return ferry trip combined with some running or walking on Staten Island makes for an excellent day's outing.

Exit the ferry terminal, bearing left. After clearing the bus plaza, admire the historic Borough Hall across the street but go immediately left down Borough Place. This takes you to the pedestrian area called North Shore Esplanade. There are many old, somewhat decrepit buildings here but there is a project in place to restore them. We expect that in due course this area will become a very popular pedestrian precinct.

Follow the path along the water. It runs into Murray Hulbert Avenue, a quiet street. Go past the George Cromwell Recreation Center, located

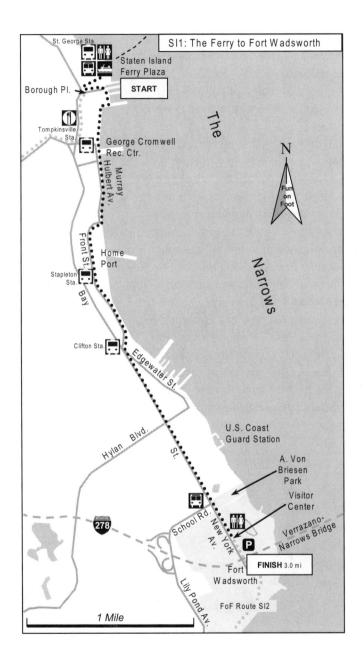

SI1: The Ferry to Fort Wadsworth

St. George Sta.

Staten Island Ferry Plaza

Borough Pl.

START

Tompkinsville Sta.

George Cromwell Rec. Ctr.

Murray Hulbert Av.

The

N

Fun on Foot

Front St.

Home Port

Stapleton Sta.

Bay

Narrows

Clifton Sta

Edgewater St.

U.S. Coast Guard Station

Hylan Blvd.

St.

A. Von Briesen Park

Visitor Center

278

School Rd.

New York Av.

Verrazano-Narrows Bridge

P

FINISH 3.0 mi

Fort Wadsworth

Lily Pond Av.

FoF Route SI2

1 Mile

FUN ON FOOT IN NEW YORK

on one of the old piers. The street becomes Front Street. Continue past the Home Port facility, the defunct Naval base in redevelopment. The street then curves back away from the water to intersect Bay Street, near the Clifton station of the Staten Island Railway. Edgewater Street joins Bay Street here.

You have a choice of following Bay Street or Edgewater Street south. Neither is very attractive, so we recommend the shorter route, Bay Street.

You come to Von Briesen Park on the left. There is little point entering that park since there is no exit from it on the water side, so continue straight ahead on Bay Street. Enter the gate into the Fort Wadsworth Gateway National Recreation Area, where the street changes name to New York Avenue. Continue on to the visitor center, a little before the enormous approach structure of the Verrazano-Narrows Bridge.

Fort Wadsworth is one of the nation's oldest military sites. The visitor center has interesting informational displays and you can obtain maps here. There are also restrooms. Note that the visitor center is closed Mondays and Tuesdays.

From this point you can connect directly to route SI2 (South and Midland Beaches). If you want to return to the ferry terminal, either reverse this route on foot or catch the S51 bus at Bay Street and School Road. Back at the ferry terminal, if you want a food or beverage break before catching the ferry, there is a bar/restaurant, Karl's Klipper, about two blocks south of the ferry terminal on Bay Street.

South and Midland Beaches

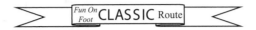

Distance	3.3 miles one way (Route SI2)
Comfort	2.5 miles of this route are on a beach boardwalk or paved multiuse trail along the beachfront. The remainder is along quiet streets inside Fort Wadsworth. Expect plenty of other pedestrians the entire route. Mostly good for inline skating.
Attractions	This route involves outstanding running or walking conditions along a scenic ocean beachfront.
Convenience	Start at Fort Wadsworth, which can be reached from the Saint George ferry terminal via route SI1 (The Ferry to Fort Wadsworth) or the S51 bus. Finish at the south end of Midland Beach where you can catch the S51 bus back to the ferry terminal. You may want to vary the start and finish points to better suit your own transport arrangements. There is ample parking at various points along the beaches. Also, the S51 bus runs the length of these beaches on Father Capodanno Boulevard.
Destination	The destination is the beach. There are services at various locations in season.

The beaches along the mid-east coast of Staten Island are popular, beautiful, and well maintained. They have a paved multiuse trail their entire 2.5-mile length, with a pedestrian-only boardwalk paralleling the trail for 1.4 of those miles.

One example of using the boardwalk for running is the Memorial Day Four-Mile Race, which starts and finishes near Sand Lane and Father Capodanno Boulevard. It uses the latter street for its outbound and the boardwalk for its return. Nola and I have run that race and agree it is one of the loveliest of that distance to be found in the city.

The majority of the people using these beaches and the trail are locals, who drive and park here. However, it is possible to get here without a vehicle, even from Manhattan. Our previous route showed how to get to Fort Wadsworth from the ferry terminal on foot. Once there, it is only 0.8 miles to the start of the boardwalk, so we chose to describe this route starting there.

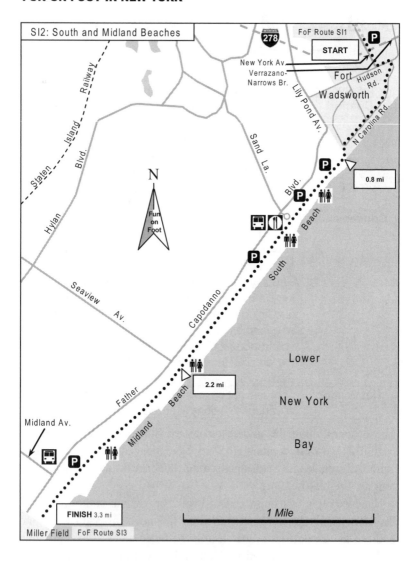

From the Fort Wadsworth visitor center on New York Avenue, go under the Verrazano-Narrows Bridge approach, noting that you are literally below the starting stage of the New York City Marathon. Continue to the end of New York Avenue. Go left into Hudson Road and right into North Carolina Road. This is a very quiet street, used as much by pedestrians as by vehicles.

Where North Carolina Road swings inland, there is a trailhead for a paved multiuse trail called the Shore Path Connector, part of the New York City Greenway system.

The trail leads to the north edge of South Beach, where the boardwalk starts, paralleling the paved bike trail. There is parking here and at several other points along the trail.

Where Sand Lane meets the shore there is a pavilion with restrooms and other services. This is also the location of the South Fin Grill, the only bar/restaurant on this route. The restaurant is quite up-market, but the bar is more informal. The food is excellent, including a Sunday brunch offering.

At Seaview Avenue the boardwalk ends but the paved multiuse trail continues. You are now entering Midland Beach. Continue to the end of Midland Beach and the end of the paved trail, at the boundary of Miller Field.

You have various options as to what to do next, including heading back on foot to where you parked. If you do not have a vehicle, the easiest way to get back to the ferry terminal is to backtrack a short distance to Midland Avenue and catch a northbound S51 bus at Midland

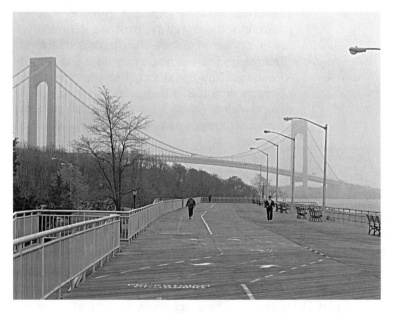

The South Beach Boardwalk with its Bridge Backdrop

Avenue and Father Capodanno Boulevard. Another good option is to continue on to Miller Field and work your way up to the New Dorp Staten Island Railway station, with several choices of wind-down food or beverage places on the way. See route SI3 (Miller Field) for more details of the last option.

Miller Field

Distance	Various (Route SI3)
Comfort	There is a 1.8-mile loop on a paved path around the park. Optionally connect 0.7 miles to or from the Long Island Railway station via the sidewalk of a busy road, or join the Midland Beach boardwalk. Expect many other pedestrians the entire route. Not recommended for inline skating.
Attractions	This route connects the south end of the Midland Beach boardwalk to a rail station and bar/restaurant strip. Miller Field is also of historic interest as a very early military airfield. There are some unrestored original facilities still there.
Convenience	Start and/or finish at the south end of Midland Beach or the New Dorp Staten Island Railway station. You can treat this park as a local loop, or as a connection to route SI2 (South and Midland Beaches). There is ample parking in and around the park. You can also get to and from Saint George via the S78 bus, or to and from Staten Island Mall or Bay Ridge in Brooklyn via the S79 bus. Both buses run along Hylan Boulevard, close to Miller Field.
Destination	There are several bars and restaurants along New Dorp Lane between Miller Field and New Dorp station.

Miller Army Airfield was constructed between 1919 and 1921 as one of the nation's first coastal air defense facilities. In 1973 the National Parks Service acquired it. Today it is primarily a large recreational park, occupied almost entirely by sporting fields.

The only visible remnants of the original airfield are Hangar #38 and the Elm Tree Beacon in the south corner of the park. The Elm Tree Beacon was a light station used by coastal shipping until it was

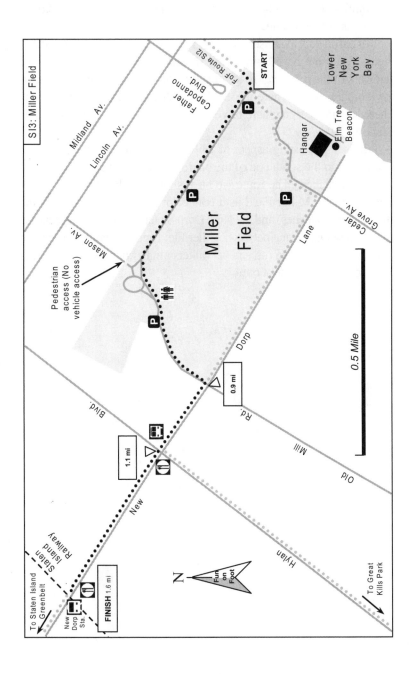

SI3: Miller Field

Lower New York Bay

START

Elm Tree Beacon

Hangar

Father Capodanno Blvd.

For Route SI2

Midland Av.

Lincoln Av.

Mason Av.

Pedestrian access (No vehicle access)

Miller Field

Cedar Av.

Grove Av.

Dorp Lane

0.5 Mile

0.9 mi

Old Mill Rd.

1.1 mi

Blvd.

New

Staten Island Railway

To Staten Island Greenbelt

New Dorp Sta.

FINISH 1.6 mi

Hylan

To Great Kills Park

N

Fun on Foot

decommissioned in 1924. Neither of these structures has been restored, so there is not a great deal to see here.

For the on-foot exerciser, there are various ways you might use Miller Field. You can run a 1.8-mile loop around the sporting fields using the sidewalk of the perimeter road for the south leg and internal park roads for the other legs. There is very little vehicle traffic to concern you. There is ample parking here or you can travel here by bus or the Staten Island Railway.

Another interesting aspect of Miller Field is that it connects at its east corner to the south end of the boardwalk and trail along South and Midland Beaches. The route we have shown on the map as a dotted black line uses Miller Field as a connector between route SI2 (South and Midland Beaches) and the New Dorp Staten Island Railway station. Along New Dorp Lane between Miller Field and the station are several restaurants and bars so runners or walkers might find this an interesting place to finish an on-foot outing.

Great Kills Park

Distance	4.2 miles out and back (Route SI4)
Comfort	An out-and-back route along an excellent quality paved multiuse trail. There is virtually no vehicle traffic to concern you. You can vary this route with some unpaved trail segments. Expect plenty of other pedestrians the entire route. Good for inline skating.
Attractions	A very pleasant environment, close to the shore, without vehicle incursions. Plenty of fresh air.
Convenience	Start and finish at the park entrance at the intersection of Buffalo Street and Hylan Boulevard. There is parking here or use any bus running along Hylan Boulevard, including buses from Saint George ferry terminal, Staten Island Mall, or Bay Ridge in Brooklyn. It is 0.7 mile on foot to the Bay Terrace Staten Island Railway station.
Destination	No specific destination.

Great Kills Park is a combination of nature preserve and recreation area. Its main attraction for on-foot exercisers is a 2.1-mile paved multiuse trail from the park entrance to the tip of Crooke's Point. We feature the out-and-back on that trail, assuming a start at the park entrance where there is parking.

Follow the trail to the next parking area. After that parking area, Bulkhead Road heads off to the right. If you want a trail map, you can get one from the Field Station on Bulkhead Road. Continue to the end of the next parking area, past the Beach Center and adjacent to the bathing beach. At the end of that parking area there is a road barrier limiting vehicles to permit holders only. Pedestrians can continue out on the trail to the tip of Crooke's Point. On the point there are also several unpaved trails to explore.

Another option, if you want to venture into the nature reserve part of the park, is as follows. Proceed out on the paved trail roughly a mile to the intersection with a sign to the boat launch ramp. Go right, through the boat launch car park to the shore of Great Kills Harbor. Go counterclockwise around the harbor using paths and edges of unpaved roads. Pass the intersection with Bulkhead Road and continue to the

---

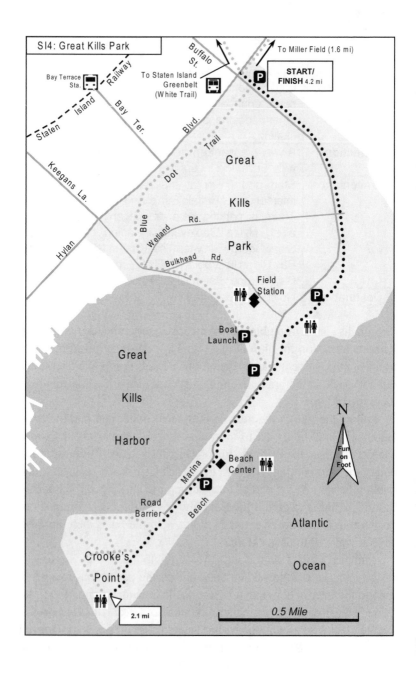

SI4: Great Kills Park

Buffalo St.

To Miller Field (1.6 mi)

To Staten Island Greenbelt (White Trail)

START/ FINISH 4.2 mi

Bay Terrace Sta.

Staten Island Railway

Bay Ter.

Keegans La.

Blvd.

Dot Trail

Great

Kills

Park

Blue Wetland Rd.

Bulkhead Rd.

Field Station

Boat Launch

Great

Kills

Harbor

Marina

Beach Center

Road Barrier

Beach

Crooke's

Point

2.1 mi

Hylan

N

Fun on Foot

Atlantic

Ocean

0.5 Mile

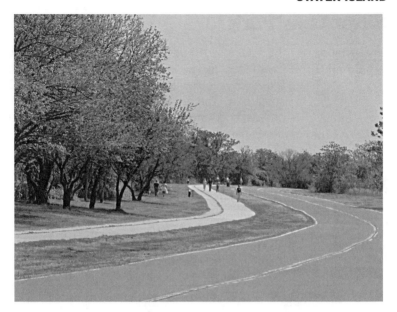

The Popular Paved Trail in Great Kills Park

intersection with Wetland Road. At this intersection there is a trailhead on the right for the Blue Dot Trail.

The Blue Dot Trail is a nature preserve trail, mainly intended for hiking and nature appreciation, but it is mostly OK for trail running. It leads back to the parking lot at the park entrance. The total length of the loop just described is roughly 2.2 miles.

You can connect your outing in Great Kills Park with Miller Field, as described in route SI3 (Miller Field). However, at present the best way to connect is via the sidewalk of Hylan Boulevard or nearby suburban streets for a distance of roughly 1.6 miles. We look forward to a nice seaside trail from Miller Field to Great Kills Park one day.

Silver Lake Park

Distance	1.5 miles loop (Route SI5)
Comfort	There is a mostly level paved trail around the lake, with an option to use other paved trails with some hills. There is no vehicle traffic in the park on weekends and holidays. Expect plenty of other pedestrians the entire route. Not suitable for inline skating.
Attractions	A very pleasant urban park setting.
Convenience	Start and finish at the intersection of Victory Boulevard and Forest Avenue. You can get here on-foot from the Saint George ferry terminal, 1.3 miles away via Bay Street and Victory Boulevard. Alternatively, take the S48, S61, S62, or S66 bus. There is usually parking to be found in the streets surrounding the park.
Destination	No specific destination.

Silver Lake was originally a spring-fed body of water. In the 19th century it was a popular recreational site and in the early years of the 20th century the lake and its immediate surrounds were acquired by the state for use as a park. The lake was subsequently converted to a reservoir as part of the Catskill water supply system. Much of the land that constituted the 209-acre park was then subsumed into a public golf course and continues in that role today.

The parkland close to the reservoir has many trees and pleasant landscaping, and is available for outdoor recreation purposes, including on-foot exercise. There is an excellent, level paved trail around the reservoir plus some more hilly terrain with paved trails on its east side.

We assume a start at the intersection of Forest Avenue and Victory Boulevard. To get here, you can walk or run from the ferry terminal or Tompkinsville Staten Island Railway station via Bay Street and Victory Boulevard. The area you pass through is generally light commercial and not very attractive, but it is only 1.3 miles from the ferry terminal (1.0 mile from the rail station). Alternatively you can take any Victory Boulevard bus from the ferry terminal, or drive and park in the streets around the park.

The most popular on-foot loop is the loop closest to the lake. From the corner, take the path down the slope to the lake edge. The loop length is 1.2 miles and add 0.3 mile to get to and from the street intersection. Go around either way and do as many loops as you want. On a nice day, you will likely pass many other on-footers here, but there is enough room not to feel crowded.

The western edge of this route follows the road called Silver Lake Park Road. There is a paved trail along that road and, furthermore, the road is closed to vehicles on weekends and holidays.

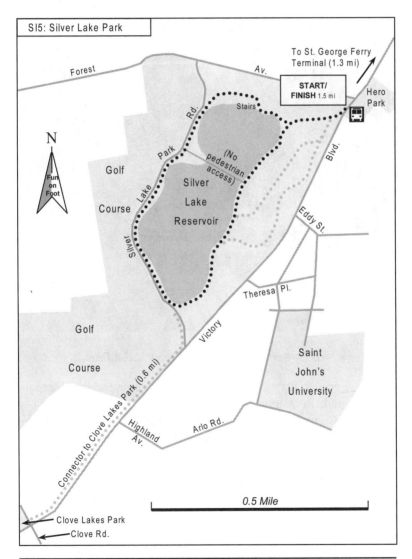

VARIATION

On the east side of the park, there is a substantial rise in the land from the lakeshore up to Victory Boulevard, and there are several trails in this part of the park. If you want to include some hills in your exercise outing, go up the rise and run or walk at the higher level of the park paralleling Victory Boulevard. This will add distance to your loop, as well as the gradients. It is generally very pleasant up here, thanks to some beautiful landscaping work.

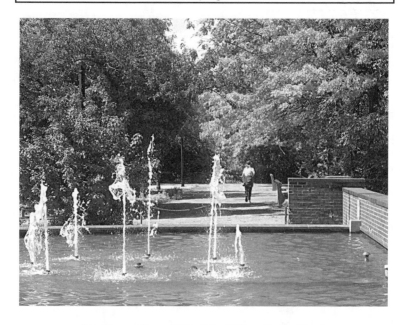

An Upper Level Trail in Silver Lake Park

If you need food or a beverage after your exercise here, you can go to the Veranda Restaurant at the golf club on Victory Boulevard.

If you want to experience Clove Lakes Park as well as Silver Lake Park in the one outing, you can connect from the southern end of Silver Lake Reservoir via the sidewalk of Victory Boulevard to the east corner of Clove Lakes Park. This is where route SI6 (Clove Lakes Park) starts.

Clove Lakes Park

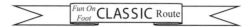

Distance	Various (Route SI6)
Comfort	Our featured route uses mostly paved trails, with some unpaved sections and some sections where there are few other pedestrians. You can alternatively do a simple loop of two or three lakes, entirely on paved trails with plenty of other pedestrians around. Not suitable for inline skating.
Attractions	This is a beautiful park with a nicely landscaped environment around the lakes, with options to go into forested areas.
Convenience	Start and finish at the intersection of Victory Boulevard and Clove Road. You can get here on foot from the Saint George ferry terminal, 2.5 miles away, or take the S61, S62, or S66 bus. There is usually parking to be found in the streets surrounding the park.
Destination	No specific destination, but there are fast food joints on Victory Boulevard if you are hungry.

This 198-acre park occupies a narrow valley and brook which, owing to various damming activities over the years, now takes the form of three linked lakes. The land was acquired as a city park in the 1920s and has been progressively developed for recreational purposes since then. Today it is a very beautiful park with some excellent on-foot trails. The landscaping includes some quaint stone-arch bridges.

You have many choices of route here. The most popular is a simple loop of the string of three lakes. We shall cover that but also feature a longer and more challenging route.

We assume a start at the intersection of Victory Boulevard and Clove Road. To get here, you can walk or run from the ferry terminal via Bay Street and Victory Boulevard. It is 2.5 miles from the ferry terminal on the streets but you should divert through Silver Lake Park, which adds a little distance—see route SI5 (Silver Lake Park). Alternatively you can take any Victory Boulevard bus from the ferry terminal, or drive and park in the streets around the park.

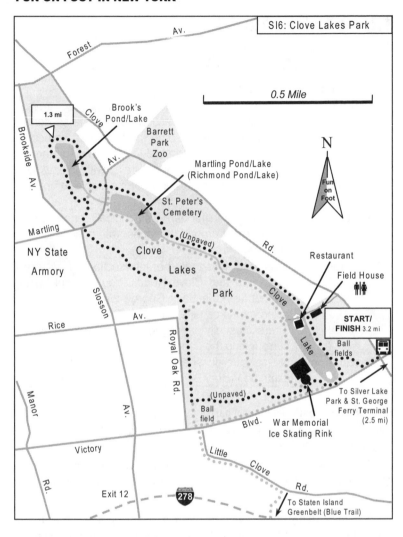

S16: Clove Lakes Park

From Victory Boulevard, follow a paved trail into the park to get to the edge of Clove Lake. Head north, counterclockwise around the lake to the first bridge. On the right is the Field House, an impressive stone building, where there are restrooms. On the left is the Lake Club restaurant, probably a little too up-market for the average on-foot exerciser.

Continue around Clove Lake (paved trail either side) to its north end, where there is a bridge across the creek. Then follow the creek

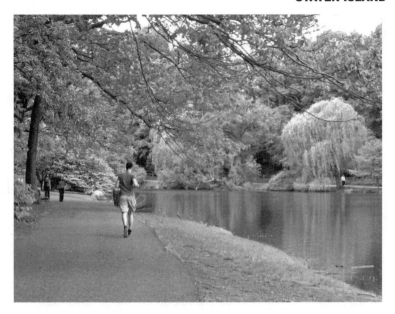

A Typical Clove Lakes Park Trail

further north—the west side of the creek has a paved trail; the east side has an earth trail and is used much less.

You then come to Martling Lake (also known as Martling Pond, Richmond Lake, or Richmond Pond) which has paved trails both sides and bridges both ends so choose whichever side you wish.

At the top end of Richmond Lake you meet the rude incursion of a trafficked road—Martling Avenue—crossing the park. On the east side of the creek, cross Martling Avenue and continue up the trail to the third lake, Brook's Lake (also known as Brook's Pond).

VARIATION

Looping the lower two lakes without going further north is a popular option and is conveniently a 1.0-mile loop. (Add 0.3 mile to connect to and from the Victory Boulevard and Clove Road intersection.)

At the south end of Brook's Lake there is a footbridge over the creek. Pass the trail to the footbridge and go up the east side of the lake on the paved trail. At the top end of the lake, cross to the west side on the footbridge there.

> **VARIATION**
> The trails continue a short distance further north on both sides of the creek but there are no more lakes and there is increasing vehicle noise so you miss nothing by turning back south here.

Head south down the west side of Brook's Lake. At the south end of the lake, you come to a trail junction with a footbridge over the creek on your left. Bear right away from the lakes.

> **VARIATION**
> At this point you can choose to go back down the lakes, making it a three-lake loop. This loop is approximately 1.4 miles. (Add 0.3 mile to connect to and from the Victory Boulevard and Clove Road intersection.

The trail away from the lakes leads to the street intersection of Martling Avenue and Slosson Avenue. Cross Martling Avenue and pick up the beautiful trail continuing into the park on the other side. Follow it straight ahead to where it becomes a trail following Royal Oak Road southward.

About 200 yards before you reach Victory Boulevard there is a well-used unpaved path heading off into the woods. Follow that path and keep heading straight at the first trail intersection, where another trail heads off to the left. The trail you are now on is not ideal underfoot—it is a little steep downhill and somewhat rocky. Continue straight ahead, hearing the sounds of Victory Boulevard not far away on your right. This short, rocky trail then meets a paved trail. Follow that paved trail to the right.

> **VARIATION**
> You can avoid the unpaved trail by continuing on the paved trail following Royal Oak Road. That trail leads to Victory Boulevard, where you can go left along the sidewalk to rejoin our main route by the War Memorial Ice Skating Rink. While this option is better underfoot, the nearby vehicle traffic detracts from its appeal.

Follow the paved trail to the War Memorial Ice Skating Rink. Go past the rink to the edge of Clove Lake and back to our starting point. There are fast food joints around here, if you need a snack after your exercise.

Staten Island Greenbelt

Distance	Various (Route SI7)
Comfort	The only wide, formed trail in the Greenbelt is the partly built Bicycle Path, which has a crushed stone surface and is very good underfoot for runners. Other Greenbelt trails are hiking/nature trails, most being suitable for the dedicated trail runner, but conditions vary with the season. All trails are blazed. Expect to pass other pedestrians on the better trails, but crowding is unlikely to be a problem. Not suitable for inline skating.
Attractions	A breathtaking escape from the city scene into wilderness. There is an enormous variety of natural environments, including woodlands, wetlands, and meadows. Plant and wildlife species abound.
Convenience	Start and finish at the Greenbelt Nature Center, off Rockland Avenue at Brielle Avenue. Alternatively, start and finish at High Rock Park, at the end of Nevada Avenue, off Rockland Avenue. You can drive and park at either place or take the S54 or S57 bus from local points. There are also many other points from which you might wish to access the Greenway trails.
Destination	No specific destination.

The Staten Island Greenbelt is an amazing preserve of 2,800 acres of parks and natural areas, hidden in the middle of Staten Island. There are over 30 miles of hiking and trail-running routes through this area. The Greenbelt is mostly New York City parkland, maintained by the city in conjunction with the Greenbelt Conservancy.

There is one good quality loop designed for bikes and runners. The other trails are hiking trails, which may be suitable for trail running. The longer trails are all blazed, but they are nature trails and are of varying quality, so can be difficult to follow if you have not been there before. Nevertheless, if you need some hill work for your training program, there is no better place.

For visitors the best starting point is the Greenbelt Nature Center at 700 Rockland Avenue at Brielle Avenue. The alternative is High

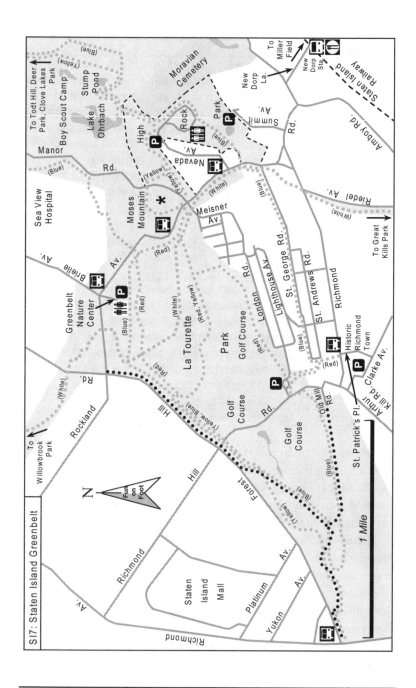

SI7: Staten Island Greenbelt

Rock Park, reachable via Nevada Avenue off Rockland Avenue, north of Richmond Road. You can pick up trail maps at either place and there are restrooms at both.

The main trails are as follows:[2]

- **Greenbelt Bicycle Path:** A groomed trail with a crushed stone surface, ideal for running. At present, 2.6 miles of the trail are under construction and will hopefully be complete by the time you read this book. This piece of trail is indicated by the dotted black line on the map. There are plans to later extend the trail into a loop, including access from the Greenbelt Nature Center. Pending completion of that loop, you can build your own loop using the initial bicycle path segment plus parts of the Red Trail (see below).
- **Blue Trail:** An easy/moderate hike, 12.3 miles one way. It stretches from near Sea View Hospital and the Greenbelt Nature Center to Deer Park via High Rock Park. From the Deer Park end, you can connect to Clove Lakes Park on foot via the street sidewalks; see Route SI6 (Clove Lakes Park).
- **White Trail:** An easy/moderate hike, 7.6 miles one way. Its southern end connects to Great Kills Park; see route SI4 (Great Kills Park).
- **Red Trail:** An easy/moderate four-mile loop trail, which starts and finishes at Historic Richmond Town, on Richmond Road at Saint Patrick's Place.
- **Yellow Trail:** A moderate/difficult trail, eight miles one-way. Its northeast end is in the Todt Hill-Emerson Hill area and it passes through Reed's Basket Willow Swamp and climbs Todt Hill here. Its southwest end is on Richmond Avenue, just south of Staten Island Mall. It passes through High Rock Park and also goes around Moses Mountain. Moses Mountain is the enormous mound of earth, now all green, that is all that remains of the hotly opposed and defeated plan by Robert Moses, the former Triborough Bridge and Tunnel Authority Chairman, to carve a parkway through this beautiful area in the 1960s.

---

2   These trail descriptions are extracted with permission from Greenbelt Conservancy materials.

Every April there is a 10K adventure race conducted here—the High Rock Challenge. The course typically uses trails in High Rock Park and extending north from there.

If you want to find a destination for a wind-down beverage or food after exercising here, there are places at the extremities of some trails but nothing central. Historic Richmond Town is a great destination for folks who like to explore historic buildings, but there is no pub or restaurant, if that is what you seek. If ending at High Rock Park, there are food and beverage places in New Dorp Lane, which is not far away and downhill all the way. There is also a Staten Island Railway station here or you can connect on foot to Miller Field and the beaches; see route SI3 (Miller Field). However, if you want to also start your outing there, be warned there is a substantial uphill climb along the street sidewalks up to High Rock Park.

More information on the Greenbelt is available from the Greenbelt Conservancy website www.sigreenbelt.org. You can also download a trail map there, or better still, pick up a copy of their printed map, available at the main trailheads.

Conference House Park

Distance	1.8 miles loop (Route SI8)
Comfort	A mixture of paved and unpaved trails. Expect other pedestrians around but not crowds. Not suitable for inline skating.
Attractions	A beautiful park by the sea with excellent quality trails. There are several historic houses nearby.
Convenience	Start and finish at the extreme end of Hylan Boulevard, at Craig Avenue. There is parking and the S78 bus stops here. The nearest Staten Island Railway station is Tottenville, about 0.7 mile north.
Destination	No specific destination.

At the southern tip of Staten Island is Conference House Park, named after the 1680-vintage historic house where the last (failed) Revolutionary War peace conference took place in 1776. This 267-acre park is beautifully maintained and has some excellent, wide running trails, some paved and some unpaved.

You can do a very pleasant 1.8-mile loop on a combination of paved and gravel trails or vary this to your taste.

Start at the very end of Hylan Boulevard where you can drive and park or take a bus. There is a visitor center here with maps and restrooms.

Head west, past the historic Conference House, towards the water of Arthur Kill, where there is a lovely pavilion structure giving relaxing views westward to the New Jersey shore. From here, head south down either of the well maintained gravel trails. These trails meet up and continue down to the western extremity of Billop Avenue. There is a short path to the water here and at its end is the "South Pole," a marker post indicating the most southerly point of New York State.

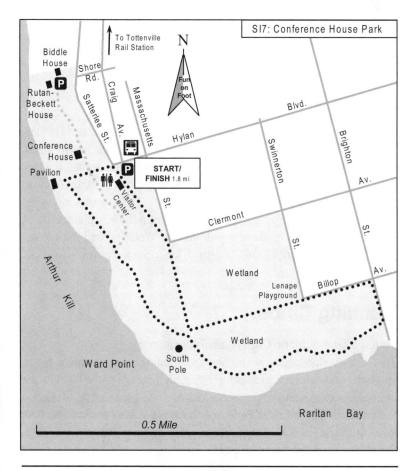

Continue on the gravel trail, over the little creek bridge and past the bird-viewing structure. The park map shows a northbound trail branch up from here through the wetland area but the condition of that trail can be questionable.

Continue to where the trail emerges on Brighton Street. Go up this quiet street and turn left into Billop Avenue. This leads you back to a park entrance, near the Lenape Playground. Follow the paved trail along the now-closed section of Billop Avenue. Turn right with the paved trail and then bear left onto the angled trail back to the visitor center.

When you have had enough exercise, you can relax and enjoy the pleasant environment around the pavilion, or take in the historic houses in the northern part of the park. If you are seeking a restaurant or bar, go north up Craig Avenue a little over a half-mile to Main Street. The Tottenville Staten Island Railway station is near here, with service to the Saint George ferry terminal.

Other Routes

Wolfe's Pond Park is on the island's southeast shore, about halfway between Great Kills Harbor and Conference House Park. It is a popular, scenic park with a one-mile paved trail plus some nature trails. To drive here, take Hylan Boulevard, turn towards the sea at Cornelia Avenue, and proceed to the park entrance on the right. There is parking in the park. It is also possible to get here on-foot from the Hueguenot Staten Island Railway station, about a mile away. Wolfe's Pond Park is the venue for the Staten Island Athletic Club's Saint Patrick's Day 5K race.

Running Clubs

Staten Island Athletic Club (statenislandac.com)
This club welcomes new members, including men, women, teens, children, and families, and athletes of all fitness levels. There are monthly meetings and open, free, clocked three-mile fun run/walks on Saturdays in Clove Lakes Park; see the website for details. The club hosts the Saint Patrick's Day 5K race in Wolfe Pond Park.
Email: Refer to "Contact Us" page of website.

7

Hudson River Jersey-Side

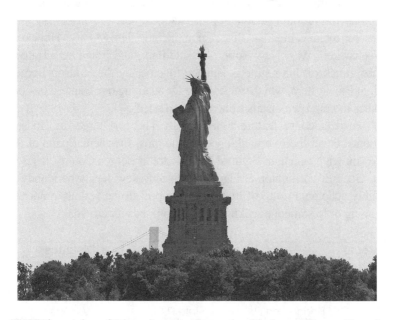

The strip of New Jersey along the Hudson River, directly across from Manhattan, is as familiar visually to most New Yorkers and visitors as are many parts of the city's boroughs. Hudson County, which accounts for the bulk of that strip, has often been referred to as New York City's sixth borough. There are numerous ways to conveniently move between this part of New Jersey and Manhattan, including the George Washington Bridge, two road tunnels, two tunnels for the Port Authority's PATH train service, and several ferry services.[1]

---

1   Chapter head photo: The rear view of the Statue of Liberty from Liberty State Park.

The New Jersey side of the Hudson is a popular dormitory area for New York City workers. It is also a well-kept secret that it is an excellent place for visitors to Manhattan to stay, with hotel rates much lower than Manhattan's and with little inconvenience penalty.

This part of New Jersey has historically been integrated with New York City from both the commercial and cultural perspective. It acted for many years as the rail transport head for goods arriving at and departing from New York Harbor. It also acted as the clearing point for many immigrants arriving from overseas and passing through the famous immigration station on Ellis Island.

The main centers in this region include Jersey City, Hoboken, Weehawken, West New York, Cliffside Park, and Fort Lee. Transit-wise, much of this region is stitched together by the Hudson-Bergen Light Rail system, which you can use for adapting our featured on-foot routes to your own distance and transport needs.

We decided to feature four routes. The first three, in Hudson County, cover the riverbank opposite the most spectacular parts of the Downtown Manhattan skyline. The fourth, in Bergen County, takes in the George Washington Bridge and adjacent New Jersey parkland—a highly adaptable route of tremendous appeal to the serious runner in training or to someone seeking escape from the city crowds.

Route	Distance
HJ1 Liberty State Park	4.1 miles loop
HJ2 Newport to Liberty State Park	3.2 miles one way
HJ3 Hoboken to Newport	3.3 miles one way
HJ4 GW Bridge and Palisades State Park	Various

The first three of these routes can be linked to each other to form longer routes. Some possibilities are:

- Starting in Newport (convenient to Manhattan via PATH train) do route HJ2, then route HJ1 (a loop of Liberty State Park), and then catch a ferry back to Manhattan; total distance 7.3 miles;

- Starting in Hoboken North (convenient to Manhattan via ferry) do routes HJ3, HJ2, and HJ1, and return to the start via Light Rail or to Manhattan by ferry; total distance 10.6 miles.

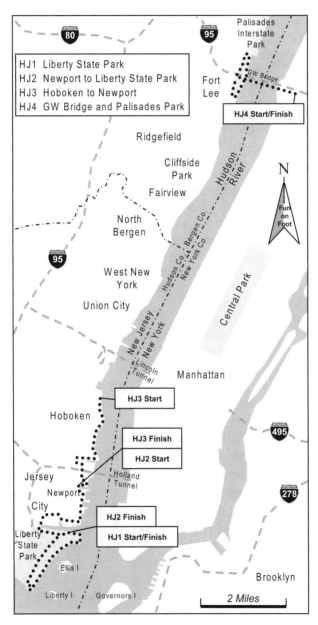

Hudson River Jersey-Side Routes

Liberty State Park

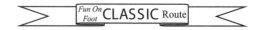

Distance	4.1 miles loop (Route HJ1)
Comfort	Excellent underfoot conditions with plenty of on-foot exercisers around. The entire route is on paved multiuse paths. Good for inline skating.
Attractions	Outstanding views of the Statue of Liberty and Ellis Island, without having to fight the crowds on the ferries. See the historic Central Railroad of New Jersey terminal and Liberty Science Center. Enjoy the fresh air, open spaces, and the unforgettable panoramic views of Downtown Manhattan.
Convenience	Start and finish at the Liberty Landing Marina, which can be conveniently reached from Manhattan by ferry. Alternatively, drive and park here, take the Hudson-Bergen Light Rail, or follow route HJ2 (Newport to Liberty State Park) from Newport in Jersey City.
Destination	See the nearby historic railroad terminal, have drinks and food at the marina restaurant, and catch a ferry back to Manhattan.

Liberty State Park is an amazing place which no on-footer should miss. It is a 1,212-acre park, comprising mostly open green space, with some spectacular views and various attractions. The park was established in the 1970s and presented as New Jersey's gift to the nation for the 1976 bicentennial celebrations.

As well as having great tourist appeal, Liberty State Park is an excellent place for on-foot exercise. There is a spectacular paved walkway the length of the waterfront, plus several trails a little inland. We chose to feature the longest loop here, which includes the walkway. There are several other trails inside this loop, allowing you to easily shorten or otherwise vary your route.

We start at the Liberty Marina, where there is a ferry service from Manhattan (not in winter) and also plenty of parking. The ferry service is called the Liberty Landing Water Taxi, and it leaves from the World Financial Center.

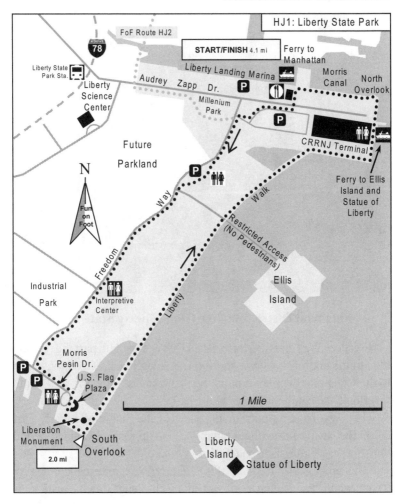

HJ1: Liberty State Park

Exit the marina area to the main road, Audrey Zapp Drive, and cross that road to the large parking area. Bear right to Freedom Way and take the paved trail to the left following that street. It takes you to the south end of the park.

VARIATION

There are several other trails through the grassed area between Freedom Way and the water. Pick your own path but be sure to go all the way down to the south corner of the park.

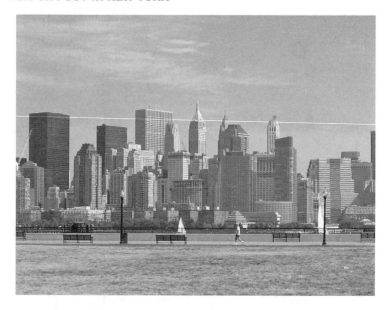

Financial District Skyline from Liberty State Park

Freedom Way ends at Morris Pesin Drive. Bear left, past the parking lots, to the end of the street and the U.S. Flag Plaza. Go right, down to the water and then left around the picnic areas. You arrive at South Overlook, the southern corner of the park.

Here you have an outstanding view of the Statue of Liberty, just 2,000 feet away, and without having to line up for an extended period with hordes of tourists to catch the ferry there.

This point is also the start of the Liberty Walk, an excellent quality paved walkway heading northeast along the length of the park. It takes you very close to Ellis Island. Ellis Island was opened in 1892 and became the nation's premier federal immigration station. In operation until 1954, the station processed over 12 million immigrant steamship passengers. The main building was restored after 30 years of abandonment and opened as a museum in 1990.

You pass a narrow bridge to Ellis Island but its use is restricted to authorized service vehicles and unfortunately we on-footers are barred from getting there that way.

Continue on the Liberty Walk to the decaying Central Railroad of New Jersey (CRRNJ) terminal. This massive railroad terminal was

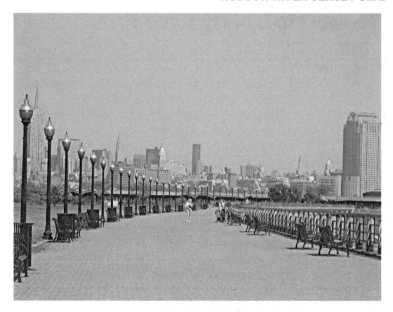

Liberty Walk

established in the late 19th century and handled 300 trains per day at its peak, around the turn of the century. It ceased operations in 1967. With restoration in mind, it is now part of Liberty State Park.

From the river side of the CRRNJ terminal you can catch a ferry to the Statue of Liberty or Ellis Island but you should obtain a ticket in advance.[2]

Keep going north along the riverbank to the North Overlook, where you have a scenic view of Downtown Manhattan. Continue on the path back to the Liberty Landing Marina area, where this route started. There is a ferry service from here to the World Financial Center at Battery Park City. There is also a restaurant and bar here, if you could use a food or beverage break while waiting for the next boat.

Another option is to go 0.8 mile up Audrey Zapp Drive to the Light Rail station, to get to other Hudson River Jersey-side destinations, including PATH rail stations to take you to Manhattan.

---

2   For more information, visit www.statuecruises.com.

Newport to Liberty State Park

Distance	3.2 miles one way (Route HJ2)
Comfort	Roughly half this route is on high quality riverside walkways and the rest follows street sidewalks. There is little vehicle cross-traffic. Expect other pedestrians around, although you might be on your own on the final part of the route. Not suitable for inline skating.
Attractions	Enjoy the unforgettable panoramic views of Downtown Manhattan. Pass the Jersey City 9/11 Memorial. Finish in historic Liberty State Park.
Convenience	Start at the Pavonia-Newport PATH station, with train service from Manhattan, or connect from route HJ3 (Hoboken to Newport). Finish at the Liberty Landing Marina with (seasonal) ferry service to Manhattan. The marina is a short walk from the Hudson-Bergen Light Rail, which connects to PATH train stations and other ferries.
Destination	Liberty State Park, with its outstanding views of the Statue of Liberty, Ellis Island, the Manhattan Financial District, and New York Harbor. Have drinks or food at the marina restaurant/bar, and catch public transit back to Manhattan.

Newport, part of Jersey City, is an amazing, newly revitalized area in what was not long ago a graveyard of rusting and rotting rail yards, warehouses, and docks. Today it is a quite impressive place, with many new, shiny high-rises and spick-and-span streets.

Newport is across the Hudson from the Financial District, and has very convenient access to Manhattan via the PATH train and ferries. It has quality hotels and restaurants and is definitely a place where New York City visitors should consider staying.

This route shows how to get to Liberty State Park from the center of Newport, a very worthwhile outing if you are staying in Newport, and even a good way to get to Liberty State Park from lower Midtown.

Start at the Pavonia-Newport PATH station on Pavonia Avenue in Newport. You can get here via PATH train from a Manhattan PATH station in 6th Avenue at 33rd, 23rd, 14th, or 9th Street, or in Christopher Street near Hudson Street in Greenwich Village. Alternatively, add this route onto route HJ3 (Hoboken to Newport).

Exit the station towards the south, and look for brass markers in the sidewalk indicating the Hudson River Waterfront Walkway. Follow these markers south, around the marina. Go past the Avalon Cove apartments. Continue south passing on your left the pier fully occupied with apartments. On your right you then pass the Plaza Two complex in the Harborside Financial Center—there is a good casual restaurant/bar here if you need food or a beverage.

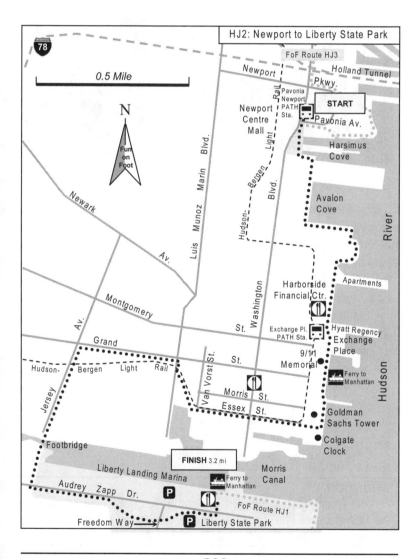

HJ2: Newport to Liberty State Park

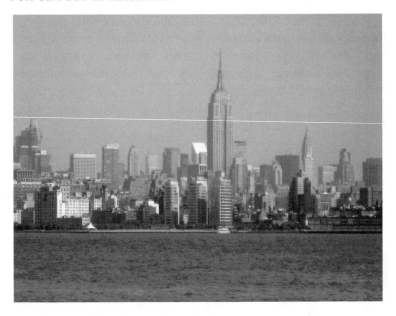

The Midtown Skyline Viewed from Newport

Pass the Hyatt Regency Hotel on the next pier, with the Exchange Place PATH station nearby. The area around here was once an enormous rail terminal, but is now all office buildings. After Exchange Place you come to the 9/11 Memorial, located directly across the river from the World Trade Center site. It includes a mesmerizing image of the view of the twin towers that used to be seen from this point.

Continue past the Goldman Sachs Tower, the tallest building in New Jersey. After this building is the famous Colgate clock—a landmark that used to grace the top of the Colgate-Palmolive warehouse that was located here until 1985. Turn inland, following Essex Street and the light rail tracks.

When you get to Washington Boulevard, you are close to some very old and interesting restaurant/pubs, mostly a block north at Morris Street. While you may not want to break your route now, remember this area for when you have a spare evening near here.

VARIATION

At Washington Boulevard you can go left from Essex Street to the Morris Canal and follow an attractive walkway there. If you do this, return to Essex Street at Van Vorst Street.

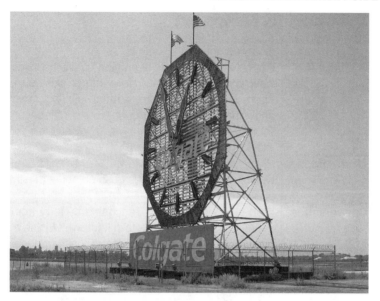

The Colgate Clock

Because of the Morris Canal basins, Essex Street ends at Van Vorst Street and you need to divert north to Grand Street to get to Liberty State Park. We found this part of the route the least attractive, due mainly to construction work at the time, but when that is complete it will be a pleasant residential area. You can use the pedestrian path along the light rail track for the first part of this diversion and then take the sidewalk up to Grand Street.

Once on the sidewalk of Grand Street, go a block west to the traffic-light intersection at Jersey Avenue. Go left here into what is mainly an industrial area. However, there is a secret at the end of this street—a footpath across a little pedestrian bridge that takes you directly into the north end of Liberty State Park.

The path from this back-door bridge leads to Audrey Zapp Drive, with the Liberty Park Science Center over to your right. Go left on the paved multiuse path along the south side of Audrey Zapp Drive. Cross Freedom Way and continue to the Liberty Landing Marina. From here you can follow route HJ1 (Liberty State Park) to see the attractions of the park. You can also get food and beverages here and (in season) take a ferry to Manhattan.

Hoboken to Newport

Distance	3.3 miles one way (Route HJ3)
Comfort	Roughly half this route is on high quality riverside walkways and the rest follows street sidewalks. There is little vehicle cross-traffic. Expect other pedestrians around, although you might be on your own in parts of the route. Not suitable for inline skating.
Attractions	Enjoy the panoramic views of Midtown and Downtown Manhattan, plus fresh air and a mostly pleasant environment.
Convenience	Start in Hoboken North, reachable by ferry from the pier at 38th-39th Streets in Midtown. Finish at the Pavonia-Newport PATH station, with frequent train service back to Manhattan. The start and finish points are also convenient to the Hudson-Bergen Light Rail.
Destination	End in Newport, Jersey City's exciting new development area, across the river from Manhattan's Financial District. There are many restaurants and bars here and convenient rail transport to Manhattan.

The Hoboken shore is a comparatively new community, across the Hudson from Midtown. It has a lovely riverfront environment, ideal for on-foot exercise. You can connect on-foot from Hoboken to Newport in Jersey City via the route described here.

Our route starts at 14th Street on the riverfront. This is at the Jersey-side dock for the ferry from the 38th-39th Streets pier in Midtown. Start immediately on the waterfront pedestrian path heading south. Hoboken North is mainly residential, with all the trappings of a young, affluent, family-oriented population. Expect to encounter many mothers out walking their children. (When we were last there, some major construction projects detracted from the environment, but they should be completed soon enough.)

Go down to Frank Sinatra Park, where there are restrooms and a café. Then continue along the foreshore to Pier A, where you can run or walk a loop of the park that occupies the pier. Admire the excellent views of the Midtown skyline.

Continue to the rail station where the riverside trail ends. If necessary, you could catch a PATH train to Manhattan or the Hudson-Bergen Light Rail here.

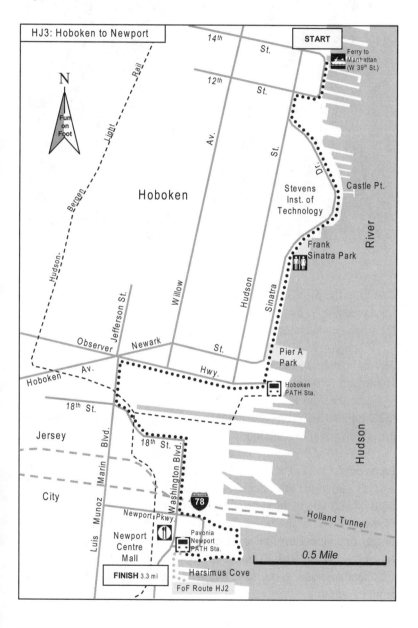

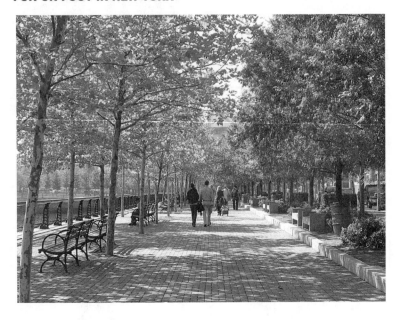

Hoboken Riverside Walk

Go to the right, on the street sidewalk of Observer Highway. It is not a pretty street but it actually provides good running conditions, since there are few vehicles and no cross streets to slow you down.

When you reach the six-way intersection where Newark Street and Jefferson Street connect from the right, go left on the sidewalk of Marin Boulevard. Go under the tracks into Jersey City.

Take the first left into 18th Street. Follow the road around into Washington Boulevard. Continue to Newport Parkway, noting that you are passing over the entrance to the Holland Tunnel.

Turn left on Newport Parkway and continue straight ahead into the entrance to the Hudson River Waterfront Walkway. Follow this walkway around to the little LeFrak Lighthouse. Continue on the walkway until it leads you to the sidewalk of Pavonia Avenue and to the Pavonia Newport PATH train station. You can catch a PATH train back to Manhattan, or continue on-foot to Liberty State Park via route HJ2 (Newport to Liberty State Park). If you want food or a beverage before moving on, there are some good restaurant/bars across Washington Boulevard from the station.

GW Bridge and Palisades Park

Distance	Various (Route HJ4)
Comfort	This route combines 1.4 miles each way on the bridge walkway with 1.9 miles (or more) in the park. The bridge walkway is shared with bikes but expect many other pedestrians too. The park loop is rugged, with some steeper sections; you will likely encounter other pedestrians on a nice day. Not suitable for inline skating.
Attractions	Outstanding views of Manhattan and plenty of fresh air on the bridge walkway. In the park, experience total escape from vehicles and crowds, with very pleasant scenery. You can visit Fort Lee Historic Park.
Convenience	Start and finish at W 178th Street and Fort Washington Avenue, on the west side of the George Washington Bus Station. This is close to the 175th Street and 181st Street stations on the 1-train subway line.
Destination	No specific destination, but there are many food and beverage places near the nominal end point.

This route is particularly important since it provides a unique opportunity to get into a large park in a wilderness environment, directly on foot from Manhattan. Even if you do not want to run on steeper and wilder trails, it can be an exhilarating outing just crossing the George Washington Bridge and sampling the lower end of Palisades Interstate Park. The massive George Washington Bridge carries the Interstate-95 traffic between New York and New Jersey, but is also a popular place for pedestrians and cyclists.

Start at W 178th Street and Fort Washington Avenue, easily reached by the 1 train or bus to the George Washington Bus Station. Follow W 178th Street west to near its end where you find a ramp heading up to the left in a loop. It takes cars, bikes, and pedestrians to the upper level of the bridge.

The pedestrian and bike way, on the south side of the bridge, gives great views of Midtown and Downtown Manhattan, if visibility is good. Expect lots of bikes but, on a nice day, expect lots of pedestrians too. It is a spectacular crossing with beautiful views and refreshing winds.

These factors compensate for the invasive noise of the nearby vehicle traffic.

The New Jersey end of the pedestrian and bike way exits onto the sidewalk of Hudson Terrace. We suggest going to the right (north). To

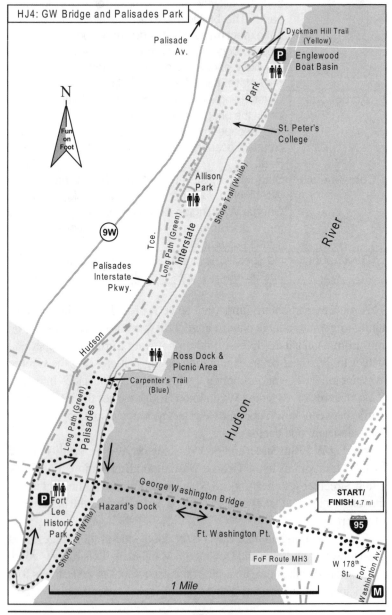

HJ4: GW Bridge and Palisades Park

Palisade Av.

Dyckman Hill Trail (Yellow)

Englewood Boat Basin

St. Peter's College

Park

N

Fun on Foot

Allison Park

Shore Trail (White)

9W

Tce.

Long Path (Green)

Interstate

River

Palisades Interstate Pkwy.

Hudson

Ross Dock & Picnic Area

Carpenter's Trail (Blue)

Long Path (Green)

Palisades

Hudson

George Washington Bridge

Fort Lee Historic Park

Hazard's Dock

Shore Trail (White)

Ft. Washington Pt.

START/ FINISH 4.7 mi

95

FoF Route MH3

W 178th St.

Fort Washington Av.

M

1 Mile

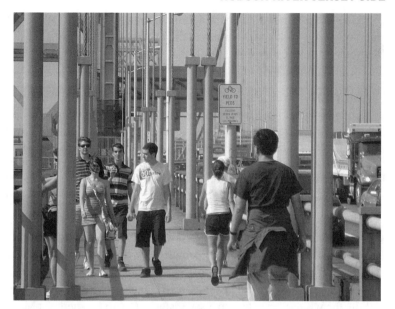

George Washington Bridge Pedestrian and Bike Way

the left is Fort Lee Historic Park, where you can pick up a trail map of Palisades Interstate Park if the visitor center is open.

Go right under the bridge approach to gain access to Palisades Interstate Park. This park occupies the bank of the Hudson and the nearby cliffs for about 12 miles, with the George Washington Bridge being close to the southern end. There are about 30 miles of hiking trails in the park. The main trails are the Long Path (green-blazed), which runs the length of the park on the top of the cliffs, and the Shore Trail (white-blazed) which runs along the riverbank. There are several short, generally steep trails that link those two main trails. Apart from near the north end of the park, the Long Path and Shore Trail are moderately level. The Long Path can be rocky underfoot and is generally less suited to running than the Shore Trail.

We limit our coverage of the park to the south end. Our main recommended route involves a 1.9-mile loop in the park, plus 1.4 miles each way on the George Washington Bridge. We also describe how to extend the park loop by about three miles, by going further upstream.

After passing under the bridge approach, go up the stairs and over the catwalk to the start of the Long Path. The first part of this trail is graveled and in excellent shape.

After half a mile, you come to a trail junction, with a sign stating 0.9 mile to Allison Park and 1.6 miles to the Dyckman Hill Trail. Take the blue-blazed trail (Carpenter's Trail) that goes down to the water here. This trail is quite steep.

VARIATION

If you want to add on an additional three miles in the park, keep to the green-blazed trail here. Continue to the Dyckman Hill Trail, which takes you down to the riverbank near Englewood Cliffs. The Long Path is somewhat rougher along here than on the first half-mile. Once down at the riverbank, return downstream on the Shore Trail to link back to our main route near the Ross Dock.

The blue-blazed trail leads you to the riverbank immediately downstream of the Ross Dock. Go to the right here, downstream. At this point, running conditions are excellent since you can use a paved road that serves a public boat ramp—there is little vehicle traffic here.

Go under the George Washington Bridge and past the boat ramp. Follow the white-blazed trail to a set of steps. Go up to emerge at Main Street, Fort Lee. Bear right along Main Street and subsequently Hudson Terrace. You pass the Fort Lee Historic Site entrance. If the historic site visitor center is open, you might want to drop in. In Main Street, there are buses to midtown or to connect with the Hudson-Bergen light rail.

Hudson Terrace leads back to the George Washington Bridge pedestrian and bike way, which returns you to Manhattan.

Running Clubs

Hoboken Harriers (www.hoha.net)
The Hoboken Harriers Running Club, founded in 1988, is a diverse group of runners and joggers from in and around Hoboken, NJ. The Club, known as the HOHAs, provides runners with camaraderie and support as well as a social component through sponsoring various social and charitable events annually. Runners of all abilities are welcome. The club sponsors the HOHA Five-Miler in early May.
Email: jim@hoha.net

South Hudson Spiked Shoe Running Club (www.shssc.org)
A small club based in Bayonne, NJ. All levels of runners are welcome. Activities include social gatherings.
Email: Refer to website

8

Westchester

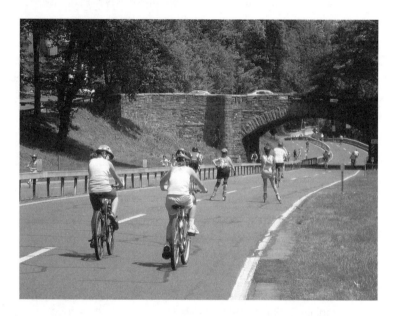

W estchester County occupies a wedge of land stretching north from the Bronx, bounded on the west by the Hudson River and on the east by Long Island Sound and the Connecticut state line. The population density is highest in the south of the county, closest to New York City—we shall focus most on that part of the county.

From an on-foot exerciser's point of view, this region has some beautiful terrain plus extensive, high quality trails. Major trail systems include:

- **The Old Croton Aqueduct:** This historic 26-mile long trail follows the Hudson River from the Croton Gorge County Park in the north to the New York City line in the south.

- **The South County and North County Trailways:** These trails use the rail bed of the now-defunct Putnam Division Railroad, which ran up the Saw Mill River Valley and northward into Putnam County.
- **The Bronx River Pathway:** This excellent trail follows the course of the Bronx River, the Metro North Harlem Line, and the Bronx River Parkway.[1]
- **The Hutchinson River Parkway Trail:** This is a series of trail segments following the Hutchinson River Parkway.

There are good north-south public transit services in the county, especially two Metro North train services that terminate at Grand Central in Midtown—the Hudson Line runs along the Hudson River bank and the Harlem Line follows the Bronx River. There is also the Metro North New Haven Line on the southeastern edge of the county following Interstate 95. East-west public transit services are harder to find, so we tend to seek on-foot routes not far from those rail services.

We decided to feature nine routes.

Route	Distance
WC1 Yonkers to Dobbs Ferry	6.0 miles one way
WC2 Dobbs Ferry to Tarrytown	4.9 miles one way
WC3 Tarrytown to Rockwood Hall	8.8 miles out/back
WC4 Rockefeller State Park Preserve	Various
WC5 Tarrytown Three-Trail Loop	10.5 miles loop
WC6 Bronxville to Scarsdale	4.6 miles one way
WC7 Hartsdale-White Plains-Valhalla	5.4 miles one way
WC8 Colonial Greenway	12.3 miles loop
WC9 Franklin D. Roosevelt State Park	Various

Some of these routes can be linked to each other to form longer routes, for example:

- Starting in Yonkers do route WC1 (Yonkers to Dobbs Ferry), then route WC2 (Dobbs Ferry to Tarrytown), and then catch a train back to Yonkers; total on-foot distance 10.9 miles;
- Starting in Bronxville do route WC6 (Bronxville to Scarsdale), follow Fox Meadow Road to Hartsdale, do route WC7 (Hartsdale-White Plains-Valhalla), and then catch a train back to Bronxville; total on-foot distance 11.5 miles.

---

1   Chapter head photo: "Bicycle Sunday" on the Bronx River Parkway (selected weekends in summer).

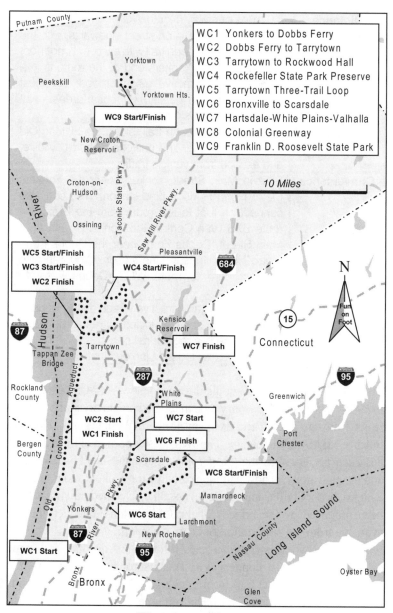

Westchester Routes

Yonkers to Dobbs Ferry

Distance	6.0 miles one way (Route WC1)
Comfort	Roughly one mile is on street sidewalks, with the remainder on an earth trail with excellent underfoot conditions. The Yonkers end of the route is in a somewhat unattractive neighborhood, but most of the route is in quality residential areas. Not suitable for inline skating.
Attractions	A very pleasant earth trail, along the historic Old Croton Aqueduct. The trail offers shade, wildlife, and escape from vehicle traffic.
Convenience	Start in Main Street, Yonkers, near the Yonkers Metro North Hudson Line station. You can also connect on foot to this route from the Bronx via route BX8 (Van Cortlandt to Yonkers). Finish in Main Street, Dobbs Ferry, near the Dobbs Ferry Metro North Hudson Line station. You can also connect here to route WC2 (Dobbs Ferry to Tarrytown).
Destination	Dobbs Ferry is an attractive village on the Hudson River, with full services including restaurants and bars. There is a regular rail service to Manhattan or to upstream Hudson Line destinations.

The Old Croton Aqueduct supplied water to New York City from 1842 to 1955. It is a buried masonry tube that relied on gravity alone to carry water from the Croton Reservoir in northern Westchester County 41 miles to Midtown Manhattan. The Westchester portion of the Aqueduct has been preserved as the Old Croton Aqueduct State Historic Park, and the path atop it is now a unique resource for walkers and runners— athletes, history buffs, and nature lovers alike. Detailed trail maps have been produced by the Friends of the Old Croton Aqueduct and are available from the www.funonfoot.com website.

Our first two Westchester routes follow the Aqueduct and some subsequent routes also connect to it. This first route covers the six-mile stretch of the Aqueduct trail from Yonkers to Dobbs Ferry. Both ends have stations on the Metro North Hudson Line, therefore you can easily complete a loop here using the train one-way if you wish. Furthermore, at both ends there are plenty of services, including restaurants and bars,

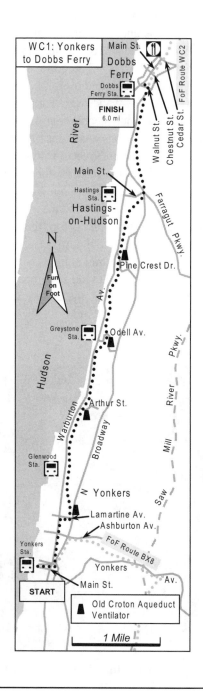

WC1: Yonkers to Dobbs Ferry

Main St.

Dobbs Ferry

FoF Route WC2

Dobbs Ferry Sta.

FINISH
6.0 mi

Walnut St.
Chestnut St.
Cedar St.

River

Main St.

Hastings Sta.

Hastings-on-Hudson

Farragut Pkwy.

N

Fun on Foot

Pine Crest Dr.

Av.

Greystone Sta.

Odell Av.

Hudson

River Pkwy.

Warburton

Arthur St.

Broadway

Saw Mill

Glenwood Sta.

N Yonkers

Lamartine Av.
Ashburton Av.

Yonkers Sta.

FoF Route BX8

Yonkers

Av.

START

Main St.

▲ Old Croton Aqueduct Ventilator

1 Mile

allowing you to easily plan an enjoyable half-day outing around this trail. Since Dobbs Ferry is unquestionably a nicer place to wait for a train than Yonkers, we describe the route ending in Dobbs Ferry.

Start in Main Street, Yonkers. There are frequent Metro North trains from Grand Central Station and a peak-hour ferry service from the World Financial Center and Wall Street. Parts of Yonkers are a little run-down but the streets our route negotiates (to get from the station to the Old Croton Aqueduct trailhead) seemed harmless enough to us.

From the rail station go up Main Street to Warburton Avenue and turn left. Pass the Philipse Manor Hall State Historic Site, Yonkers' oldest building which is now a museum. Continue up the hill to Lamartine Avenue and go right. In this street you find the inconspicuous trailhead to the Old Croton Aqueduct trail, just before the North Broadway T-junction. Follow the shady, green trail north.

We found the first part of the trail somewhat trashy and not very inviting. You might appreciate having a companion while on this Yonkers end of the trail. However, the quality of the environment improves enormously within the first mile.

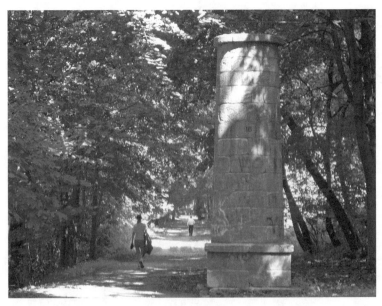

Old Croton Aqueduct Trail and Ventilator

Note the characteristic stone structures along the trail that are the ventilators of the Old Croton Aqueduct. When you reach the third ventilator (Ventilator 19), you are within easy reach of Greystone Station.

You then enter Hastings-on-Hudson. When you reach Farragut Parkway, you can leave the trail and go left down Main Street to the town center, which is mainly on Warburton Avenue. There is a Metro North station here, plus restaurants and casual food places.

Continue on the Aqueduct trail a little over a mile to Dobbs Ferry. After the trail crosses Broadway, continue on to the next street, Walnut Street, and go left down to Main Street. Our route ends here. You can either go to the left on Main Street to the Metro North station or to the right for most services. It is a very attractive village. We found an excellent food and beverage establishment, the Celtic Corner Irish Pub, at the corner of Chestnut Street and Main Street. You might want to wait for your train here (be sure to check a timetable in advance).

If you do this route in reverse, there is a selection of pubs and restaurants in Main Street, Yonkers.

Dobbs Ferry to Tarrytown

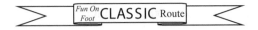

Distance	4.9 miles one way (Route WC2)
Comfort	Roughly 1.5 miles are on a street sidewalk, with the remainder on an earth trail with excellent underfoot conditions. There is considerable wildlife. Expect to pass other pedestrians but no crowds. Not suitable for inline skating.
Attractions	A very pleasant earth trail, along the historic Old Croton Aqueduct. The trail offers shade, wildlife, and escape from vehicle traffic. Pass through the magnificent Lyndhurst Estate.
Convenience	Start in Main Street, Dobbs Ferry, near the Dobbs Ferry Metro North Hudson Line station. You can also connect on foot to this route from Yonkers via route WC1 (Yonkers to Dobbs Ferry). Finish in Main Street, Tarrytown, near the Tarrytown Metro North Hudson Line station. You can also connect here to route WC3 (Tarrytown to Rockwood Hall) or WC5 (Tarrytown Three-Trail Loop).
Destination	Tarrytown is an attractive city on the Hudson River, with full services including restaurants and bars. There is regular rail service to Manhattan or to upstream Hudson Line destinations.

This is our second Old Croton Aqueduct route, starting where the previous route ended and continuing north to Tarrytown near the Tappan Zee Bridge. It is an outstanding route, regardless of which direction you do it.

We assume a start in Main Street, Dobbs Ferry. Go north up Main Street to its end at Cedar Street. Cross Cedar Street and go straight ahead, down the path to the Old Croton Aqueduct trail. Follow the trail through the Mercy College campus and past Ventilator 17.

The trail now is outstandingly beautiful. It is very green and quiet, with an English country feeling about it. We saw several deer. The trail is very popular with local runners and walkers; expect many other individuals but no crowds.

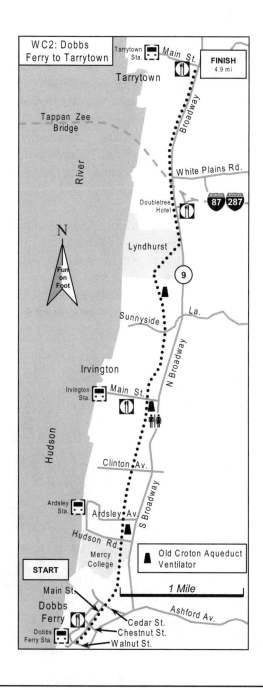

WC2: Dobbs Ferry to Tarrytown

Tarrytown Sta.

Main St.

FINISH
4.9 mi

Tarrytown

Tappan Zee Bridge

River

White Plains Rd.

INTERSTATE 87 INTERSTATE 287

Doubletree Hotel

Lyndhurst

N

Fun on Foot

9

Sunnyside

La.

N Broadway

Irvington

Irvington Sta.

Main St.

Hudson

Clinton Av.

S Broadway

Ardsley Sta.

Ardsley Av.

Hudson Rd.

Mercy College

START

Old Croton Aqueduct Ventilator

1 Mile

Main St.

Dobbs Ferry

Dobbs Ferry Sta.

Ashford Av.

Cedar St.
Chestnut St.
Walnut St.

As you approach Irvington there is a park on the east side of the trail with tennis courts and a ball field—there are convenient restrooms here. After Ventilator 16 you come to Main Street, Irvington. There are restaurants and fast food joints here and a train station at the west end of the street. You could choose to start or finish your outing here.

Continue north to Ventilator 15 where you enter the Lyndhurst Estate. Lyndhurst is a fine Gothic Revival mansion, a National Trust Historic Site, with beautifully landscaped grounds. After passing through here, the trail emerges on the sidewalk of South Broadway (Route 9).

From this point to the center of Tarrytown, the Old Croton Aqueduct is barely accessible so you should follow the sidewalk of South Broadway about 1.5 miles to the end of the route. On the way you pass the Doubletree Hotel, which has a reasonable bar and restaurant. There is also a more economical diner across the street.

Continue up South Broadway, over the New York State Throughway and past White Plains Road, to Main Street, Tarrytown. Our route ends here. Around Main Street there are several restaurants. Pubs are scarce but the Horsefeathers Restaurant further up Route 9 has a good bar. Tarrytown station is at the river end of Main Street, 0.3 mile from Route 9.

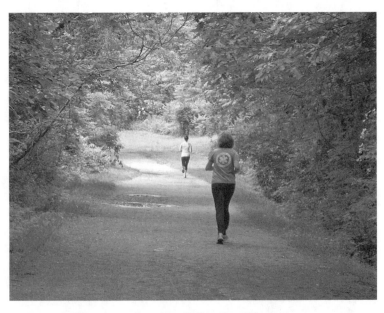

The Aqueduct Trail South of Tarrytown

Tarrytown to Rockwood Hall

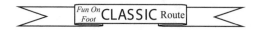

Distance	8.8 miles out and back (Route WC3)
Comfort	The entire route is on an earth trail with excellent underfoot conditions. Expect to pass other pedestrians but no crowds. Not suitable for inline skating.
Attractions	A very pleasant earth trail, along the historic Old Croton Aqueduct. The trail offers shade, wildlife, and escape from vehicle traffic. Do a loop of the magnificent and historic Rockefeller Rockwood Hall Estate, with its scenic views over the Hudson.
Convenience	Start and finish in Main Street, Tarrytown, 0.3 mile from the Tarrytown Metro North Hudson Line station. You can connect on foot from Dobbs Ferry via route WC2 (Dobbs Ferry to Tarrytown). You can also connect from here to route WC5 (Tarrytown Three-Trail Loop). Alternatively, if you are driving and parking, start and finish at the Sleepy Hollow High School.
Destination	Tarrytown is an attractive city on the Hudson River, with full services including restaurants and bars. There is a regular rail service to Manhattan or to upstream Hudson Line destinations.

The Rockefeller State Park Preserve, roughly three miles north of Tarrytown, is a marvelous resource for athletes, nature lovers, and anyone who likes spending time outdoors. The preserve has two distinct parts—the main area on the east side of Route 9 and the Rockwood Hall area on the west side of Route 9. We describe the former in the next route description (route WC4). In this route we cover the Rockwood Hall area together with the Old Croton Aqueduct trail from and to Tarrytown. This is an excellent route for athletic training, with great underfoot conditions, mostly level but with some significant grades around Rockwood Hall.[2]

---

2   Thanks to Mike Barnow of Westchester Track Club for recommending this route.

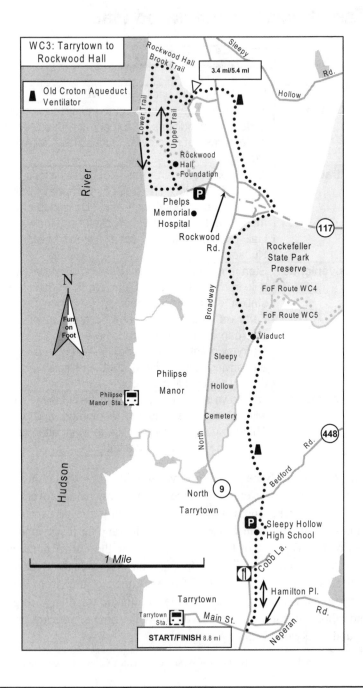

WC3: Tarrytown to
Rockwood Hall

▲ Old Croton Aqueduct
Ventilator

Rockwood Hall
Brook Trail

3.4 mi/5.4 mi

Sleepy

Rd.

Hollow

Lower Trail

Upper Trail

Rockwood
Hall
Foundation

River

P

Phelps
Memorial
Hospital

Rockwood
Rd.

117

Rockefeller
State Park
Preserve

FoF Route WC4

FoF Route WC5

N

Fun
on
Foot

Broadway

Viaduct

Sleepy

Philipse

Hollow

Manor

Philipse
Manor Sta.

Cemetery

North

448

Rd.

Bedford

1 Mile

Hudson

North

9

Tarrytown

P

Sleepy Hollow
High School

Cobb La.

Tarrytown

Hamilton Pl.

Rd.

Tarrytown
Sta.

Main St.

Neperan

START/FINISH 8.8 mi

Start at Main Street and North Broadway (Route 9). Go north up North Broadway one short block to Hamilton Place. Turn right here and pick up the Old Croton Aqueduct trail to the left about 50 yards in from North Broadway. Proceed up the Aqueduct trail to the Sleepy Hollow High School. You have to divert from the Aqueduct here, around the school that has been rudely thrown on top of the Aqueduct route. If you find the signs here confusing, ignore them and find your way around to the other side of the school, where the Aqueduct trail starts up again.

VARIATION
If you are driving and parking to do this route, a good place to park is the Sleepy Hollow High School. This reduces the distance by 0.6 mile each way, to give a total out-and-back connection plus Rockwood Hall loop distance of 7.6 miles.

Continue up the Aqueduct Trail past the Sleepy Hollow Cemetery to the viaduct over the Pocantico River. At this point you enter the Rockefeller State Park Preserve. Keep following the Aqueduct until the trail swings right just before the Route 117 highway. Cross that highway via the first pedestrian bridge over it. Bear left on the other side, to join the Aqueduct again.

Pass Ventilator 11 and cross Route 9 via the pedestrian bridge. Then take the first trail off to the left to enter the Rockwood Hall area of Rockefeller State Park Preserve.

The Rockwood Hall area is unquestionably the most beautiful part of the park. It is also the most historically interesting part and the best part for the on-foot exerciser. It is somewhat tricky to get to, which helps keep it off the tourists' route.

You enter at the top of the Rockwood Hall Brook Trail. Follow this beautiful, shady trail, which uses an Olmsted-designed carriage road, 0.4 mile down to the top of the bluff over the river. The trail follows a brook and weaves over five bridges on its way down.

At the bottom, go left on the Lower Trail along the bluff and then up the slope to the trail junction and street access point.

VARIATION
If you want to drive to the Rockwood Hall area and park, take Rockwood Road, which is the westward extension of Route 117, to the little unmarked parking lot below Phelps Memorial Hospital. Cross the street and enter the park at this point in our route.

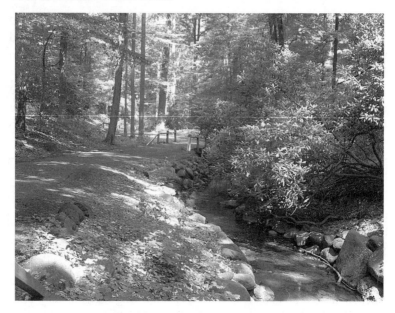

Rockwood Hall Brook Trail

Head north, keeping to the upper level of the Rockwood Hall area. This brings you via a cobblestoned carriage road to the ruins of what was Rockwood Hall, the pride and joy of the Rockefeller family, with its beautiful overlook of the Hudson River. This place is well worth seeing, and you will only see it on foot—tour buses do not drive through here.

Continue straight ahead and uphill on the Upper Trail. It leads you close to the brook but swings back towards the east. It ends at the paved road that is now just an access road to the commercial property adjacent. Turn left along the road for 100 yards to the next trailhead heading back down. (You can shortcut by using the little connecting path just below the road.) Go down the paved trail a short distance to get back to where you entered the park, the trail junction connecting to the Old Croton Aqueduct.

Return to Tarrytown, backtracking on the Old Croton Aqueduct Trail. If you seek a food or beverage break on getting back to Tarrytown, consider leaving the trail at Cobb Lane and going down to Horsefeathers on North Broadway.

Rockefeller State Park Preserve

Distance	Various (Route WC4)
Comfort	There are many trails through this park, most being shady, wide, earth trails that were originally carriage roads. There are some steeper grades but also several moderately level trails. Expect to pass plenty of other pedestrians. There are some horses. Not suitable for inline skating.
Attractions	A park with numerous well-marked trails, mostly wide and excellent underfoot. There is extensive wildlife in the park.
Convenience	Start and finish at the park's visitor center off Route 117 between Route 9 and the Taconic State Parkway. There is ample parking here but you need to pay.
Destination	No specific destination but, if you have not done so before, see the displays in the visitor center.

Rockefeller State Park Preserve is a beautiful outdoor escape area and has outstanding trails for running, jogging, or walking. Route WC3 (Tarrytown to Rockwood Hall) introduced the Old Croton Aqueduct Trail and the Rockwood Hall area on the west side of the park. In this route description, we cover the remainder of the park.

The park trails are of excellent quality, many being old carriage roads. The trail signs are outstanding, generally giving full trail names at the intersections, not just blazes. Horses are permitted on most trails and there are some restrictions on runners running in large groups.

There are many ways to craft your own trail loops. Here are three of the most popular ones:

- **Brothers' Path:** A 1.1-mile level trail around beautiful Swan Lake; convenient to the parking lot and visitor center.

- **Brook Trail - Ridge Trail - Brothers' Path Loop:** From the visitor center, go down to Swan Lake and clockwise around it to the Brook Trail. Climb up this trail through the woods, following a pleasant little brook. At the top, switch to the Ridge Trail, which initially follows the edge of an open field but later connects back to Swan Lake. Finish the loop of

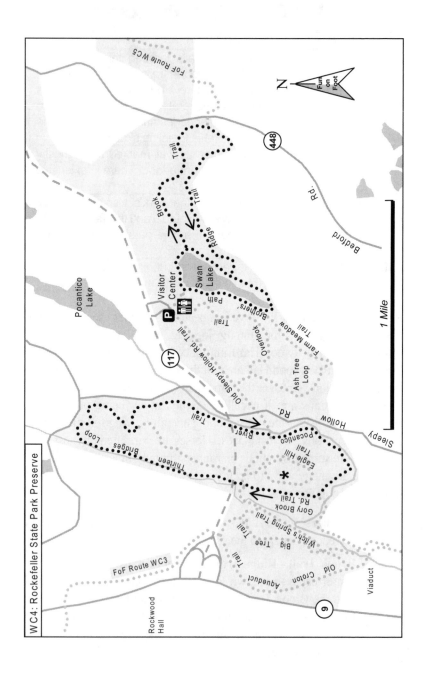

Swan Lake clockwise on the Brothers' Path. Total distance is approximately 2.5 miles.

- **Thirteen Bridges Trail - Pocantico River Trail - Gory Brook Road Trail Loop:** A more challenging loop, with some significant grades, but very beautiful and excellent underfoot. To do this loop, follow the Old Sleepy Hollow Road Trail 0.6 mile from the visitor center. Cross Sleepy Hollow Road, and cross the Pocantico River Bridge. Go south down the Pocantico River Trail, keeping to the west bank of the river. Connect to the northbound (and uphill) Gory Brook Road Trail. At the main trail junction go north under the highway on the Thirteen Bridges Loop and connect to the Pocantico River Trail southbound, returning to the Pocantico River Bridge and Old Sleepy Hollow Road Trail. The total distance is approximately four miles, not including the 0.6-mile connection each way on the Old Sleepy Hollow Road Trail.

The latter route can be easily reached on foot from Tarrytown via the Old Croton Aqueduct Trail as described in route WC3 (Tarrytown to Rockwood Hall). If doing this, leave the Aqueduct trail to the right, just before it crosses the Pocantico River on the viaduct. Follow the signs for the Pocantico River Trail. Cross the bridge over the river and join the Gory Brook Road Trail.

Tarrytown Three-Trail Loop

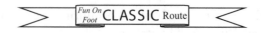

Distance	10.5 miles loop (Route WC5)
Comfort	The first 0.7 mile is on a street sidewalk and the remainder is on pedestrian earth trails and paved multiuse trails. With the exception of one short, steep climb at the east end of Rockefeller State Park Preserve, the trails are all wide and excellent underfoot, with slight to moderate grades. Expect to pass other pedestrians on most parts of the route. Not suitable for inline skating overall.
Attractions	An excellent exercise loop with few vehicle encounters, passing through a variety of terrain.
Convenience	Start and finish in Main Street, Tarrytown, 0.3 mile from the Tarrytown Metro North Hudson Line station. You can connect on foot from Dobbs Ferry via route WC2 (Dobbs Ferry to Tarrytown). Alternatively, if you are driving and parking, start and finish at the Sleepy Hollow High School.
Destination	Tarrytown is an attractive city on the Hudson River, with full services including restaurants and bars. There is a regular rail service to Manhattan or to upstream Hudson Line destinations.

Previous route descriptions have introduced the Rockefeller State Park Preserve and the Old Croton Aqueduct Trail north of Tarrytown. In this route, we add one more trail ingredient—the North County Trailway— and put all three together to give an outstanding exercise loop for anyone seeking a 10-to-11 mile excursion. For someone living or staying in the Tarrytown-Sleepy Hollow region, including students and staff of Fordham University's Tarrytown campus, this is a not-to-miss route.

The North County Trailway is a paved multiuse trail along the bed of the defunct Putnam Division of the New York Central Railroad. The "Old Put" ran between the Bronx and Putnam County until 1958. The 36 miles of the old railbed running through Westchester County have been largely converted into paved multiuse trails, in two parts: the North County Trailway on the north side of Interstate 287 and the South County Trailway on the south side of that Interstate corridor.

At Tarrytown, at the south end of the North County Trailway, there is an extension of the Trailway to connect close to central Tarrytown via a trail along the Tarrytown Lakes reservoirs. That connector makes this outstanding loop possible. The trails link together so well and the result is so exciting we declared this a Fun-on-Foot Classic Route.

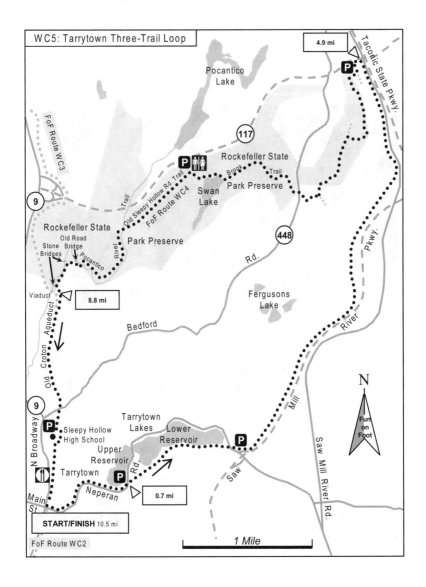

WC5: Tarrytown Three-Trail Loop

4.9 mi

Pocantico Lake

Taconic State Pkwy.

FoF Route WC3

117

Rockefeller State

Park Preserve

Brook

Trail

Old Sleepy Hollow Rd Trail

Trail

FoF Route WC4

Swan Lake

9

448

Rockefeller State

Old Road

Stone Bridge

Bridges

Pocantico

Park Preserve

River

Rd.

Viaduct

8.8 mi

Old Croton Aqueduct

Bedford

Fergusons Lake

River Pkwy.

N

9

Tarrytown Lakes

Lower Reservoir

Mill

Fun on Foot

N Broadway

Sleepy Hollow High School

Upper Reservoir

Saw Mill River Rd.

Rd

Tarrytown

Neperan

0.7 mi

Saw

Main St

START/FINISH 10.5 mi

1 Mile

FoF Route WC2

Start at the intersection of Main Street and North Broadway in Tarrytown. Follow the left sidewalk of Neperan Road uphill to Fordham University and continue to where the sidewalk ends and there is a small car park overlooking the Tarrytown Lakes Upper Reservoir. Across the road is a trailhead to the Tarrytown Lakes Extension of the North County Trailway. This stretch is flat and very pleasant and it comprises a measured mile with quarter-mile markers. It ends at Neperan Road by the reservoir dam, just before the Saw Mill River Parkway. Cross the road to the trail car park and continue on the short trail stub (there is a significant grade here) to the North County Trailway proper.

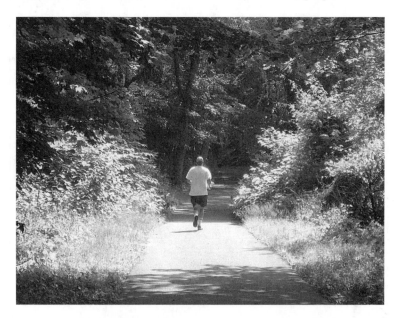

North County Trailway Tarrytown Extension

This trail initially follows the Saw Mill River Parkway and swings left to follow the Taconic State Parkway. Follow this excellent, level trail three miles to the exit point at Route 117.

Go up the exit ramp to the trail head and its small parking lot. Go around to the left into a larger, paved parking lot. At the end of the parking area is a trailhead with a sign indicating a Nature Trail to the Rockefeller State Park Preserve. At this point we should warn you that the trails for the next mile or so are not marked, and there is a serious risk of becoming lost, therefore you should follow our directions carefully.

Enter the trail system here, and at the first fork take the trail heading up the hill to the right. This is a twisty earth path. After about 200 yards it passes through a gateway in a chain wire fence to join a gravel fire road. There is a familiar trail rules sign of the State Parks organization here. You are now in the Rockefeller State Park Preserve, but a part of the preserve that was added recently and is currently deficient in trail name or directional signs. (This will likely change in due course, maybe even by the time you try this route.) Follow this fire road uphill through the woods about a half-mile to its end at a T-intersection with a wider gravel road. This intersection is distinguishable from its sign that declares that the road you just traveled has no outlet and is for hikers only. Go left about 500 yards to another T-intersection. Go left again. After about 200 yards you emerge from the woods at the top of a rise, where the road continues through pasturelands. Continue a further 200 yards to yet another T-intersection, this time with fenced pasturelands all around it. Go right and follow the road around to where it skirts Route 448 and soon afterwards arrives below a stone bridge, which takes pedestrians under the road.

Go under that bridge to enter the fully developed part of the Rockefeller State Park Preserve. From now on, all trails are very well marked with blue signs. You enter this part of the preserve at the junction of the Brook Trail and Ridge Trail. You can take either but we suggest following the Brook Trail to the right. Keep on the Brook Trail until it meets the Brothers Trail on the edge of the lake. Bear right to the visitor center, where there are restrooms and maps, both of which might be appreciated by now.

From the front of the visitor center, go left past the car park and through the gate to the Old Sleepy Hollow Road Trail. Follow this trail downhill. Go through the next gate and cross Sleepy Hollow Road, one of the very few traffic encounters of this route. Continue on across the bridge (with the brown metal handrails) over the Pocantico River. Go left down the Pocantico River Trail. It is a very pleasant trail, following the riverbank.

Keep to the west bank of the river until you meet the Gory Brook Road Trail heading off to the right. Go left across the river here and then immediately right. Cross the abandoned road near the disused road bridge. Keep to the east side of the river now, passing one stone bridge and then arriving at a second stone bridge. At this point, go left away from the river. Here you get an excellent view of the viaduct that carries the Old Croton Aqueduct across the river. Go on to where the trail joins the old road and swing right, noting the characteristic mound of the Old Croton Aqueduct on your right. Take the first path to the right up onto the Aqueduct trail.

Proceed down the Aqueduct trail, past Sleepy Hollow Cemetery, to the Sleepy Hollow High School. Divert around the school and find the trail again on the other side. Continue back to the center of Tarrytown, where this route started.

If you need a food or beverage break on getting back to Tarrytown, consider leaving the Aqueduct trail at Cobb Lane and going down to Horsefeathers restaurant and bar on North Broadway.

Bronxville to Scarsdale

Distance	4.6 miles one way (Route WC6)
Comfort	An excellent quality paved multiuse trail, with few street crossings. It is level and shady in many parts. Expect plenty of other pedestrians and cyclists. OK for inline skating.
Attractions	A very pleasant trail following the Bronx River through a series of attractive suburbs.
Convenience	Start at the Bronxville Metro North Harlem Line station near Palmer Road and Pondfield Road in Bronxville. Finish at the Scarsdale Metro North Harlem Line Station at Popham Road, Scarsdale. You can return by train. You can vary the route making use of stations at intermediate points.
Destination	Scarsdale is an attractive village on the Bronx River, with full services including restaurants and cafes. There is regular rail service to Manhattan or to northern Westchester destinations.

The next two routes involve the Bronx River Pathway, a trail along the Bronx River, generally following the Bronx River Parkway and the Metro North Harlem Line. The latter, in particular, can be very helpful to the on-foot exerciser, since it opens up the option of doing various one-way excursions, returning to the start by train.

The paved Pathway trail links together the centers of (south to north) Bronxville, Tuckahoe, Crestwood, Scarsdale, Hartsdale, White Plains, North White Plains, and Valhalla. There is one significant gap in the

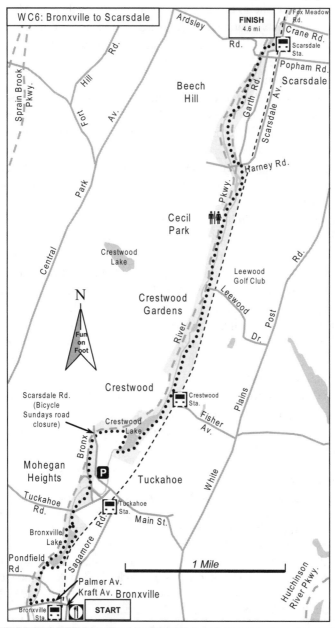

trail—roughly 1.5 miles between Scarsdale and Hartsdale. While you can cover that gap using street sidewalks, we found it convenient to split the trail at that point into two segments; hence our two distinct routes—Bronxville to Scarsdale and Hartsdale to Valhalla. All of the above centers have stations on the Metro North Harlem Line.

In summer, watch for scheduled "Bicycle Sundays." On these days the Bronx River Parkway is closed to traffic from the Westchester County Center in White Plains to Scarsdale Road near Tuckahoe. The parkway is opened up to cyclists, inline skaters, and pedestrians. For pedestrians, the roadway is no better than the Pathway trail, but you still win since the bicycle traffic mostly uses the roadway those days.

For the Bronxville to Scarsdale route, start at the Bronxville Metro North station. If you are finishing here rather than starting, there are plenty of places to wind down for food and a drink. We can personally recommend JC Fogarty's Town Tavern, an Irish pub and restaurant in Kraft Avenue, just south of the station.

Immediately north of the station is Palmer Avenue. Head west along this street and bear left into Palmer Road. Just before you reach the Bronx River Parkway, you find the trailhead to the multiuse trail on the right. Follow the trail up to Bronxville Lake, where the trail branches to go up either side of the lake. Choose whichever side you want—they meet at the north end of the lake. Skirt the edge of Tuckahoe Village.

Pass Crestwood Metro North station. After Leewood Drive you pass a tourist information booth on the edge of the parkway. There are (seasonal) restrooms here.

The trail leads to the edge of Garth Road and on to Scarsdale station. Scarsdale is a pleasant little town, with basic services but limited eating and drinking establishments. There are frequent trains connecting Bronxville and Scarsdale.

VARIATION

To connect to route WC7 (Hartsdale-White Plains-Valhalla) you need to travel about 1.5 miles on street sidewalks and unpaved trails. From Scarsdale station go north to Crane Road and a block east to Fox Meadow Road. Go north along Fox Meadow Road (or divert into the woods between Fox Meadow Road and the parkway) to Fenimore Road. Go back towards the parkway and down the steps to the fountain and gardens. Continue to Greenacres Avenue near Hartsdale Station, where route WC7 starts.

Hartsdale-White Plains-Valhalla

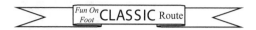

Distance	5.4 miles one way (Route WC7)
Comfort	An excellent quality paved multiuse trail, with few street crossings. It is level and shady in many parts. Expect plenty of other pedestrians and cyclists. OK for inline skating.
Attractions	A very pleasant trail following the Bronx River through a series of attractive suburbs and the center of White Plains.
Convenience	Start at the Hartsdale Metro North Harlem Line station near Hartsdale Avenue and Fenimore Road. Finish at the Valhalla Metro North Harlem Line station near the Kensico Dam Plaza. You can return by train, but will likely have to transfer at North White Plains. You can vary the route making use of stations at White Plains or North White Plains.
Destination	The Kensico Dam Plaza is an impressive place to visit, and has restrooms and snacks. From there, go 0.4 mile to the Valhalla Metro North station. At the station there is an excellent pub/restaurant to wait for your train. There is regular rail service to Manhattan or other Harlem Line destinations.

Our second Bronx River Pathway route is a beautiful route, with wildlife and a scenic environment including several stone bridges. The trail is mostly paved underfoot, with the occasional gravel stretch. There are few interruptions from road crossings.

The start and finish points are serviced by the Metro North Harlem Line, as are two intermediate points—White Plains and North White Plains. The train service connecting Hartsdale, White Plains, and North White Plains is quite frequent, with the extension to Valhalla being less frequent.

Start at the Hartsdale Metro North station. There are restrooms here. If you choose to finish rather than start here, there are some food places nearby and a nice little bar at Harrys of Hartsdale Steak House, across the street from the station.

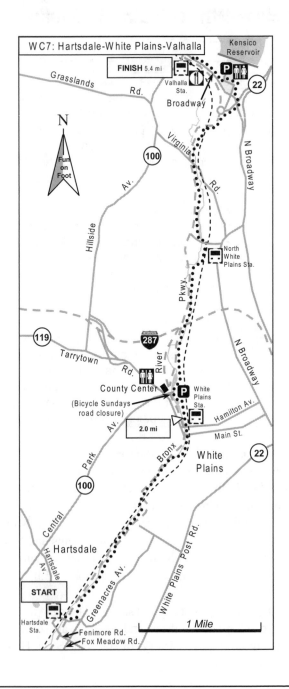

WC7: Hartsdale-White Plains-Valhalla

Kensico Reservoir

FINISH 5.4 mi

Grasslands Rd.

Valhalla Sta.

Broadway

22

N

Fun on Foot

100

Virginia Rd.

Hillside Av.

N Broadway

North White Plains Sta.

Pkwy.

119

287

Tarrytown Rd.

River

N Broadway

County Center

White Plains Sta.

P

(Bicycle Sundays road closure)

2.0 mi

Hamilton Av.

Main St.

White Plains

22

Park Av.

Bronx

Central Av.

100

Hartsdale

Hartsdale Av.

START

Greenacres Av.

White Plains Post Rd.

1 Mile

Hartsdale Sta.

Fenimore Rd.
Fox Meadow Rd.

From the station, follow Greenacres Avenue across the river and the Bronx River Parkway to the start of the Pathway trail heading north. This is a very pleasant trail which succeeds in keeping far enough away from both the parkway and the rail tracks. There is plenty of wildlife, especially ducks and geese.

The trail leads close to the center of White Plains, the county seat since 1759 and site of the Battle of White Plains fought in 1776. Go under two busy roads, Main Street and Hamilton Avenue. You can go up and follow either of these roads across the tracks into White Plains center if that is your destination. Immediately after Hamilton Avenue is White Plains station, which you can enter directly from the trail.

Continue on, skirting the large parking lot. At this point you have the opportunity to cross the parkway at a pedestrian crossing to get to the County Center. There are restrooms here.

The trail then leads to North White Plains station; there is little of interest here apart from a large commuter parking lot. One mile further on you come to the Kensico Dam plaza. The dam is enormous, making this plaza a fascinating place. There are restrooms and a snack bar here, along with a large free parking lot.

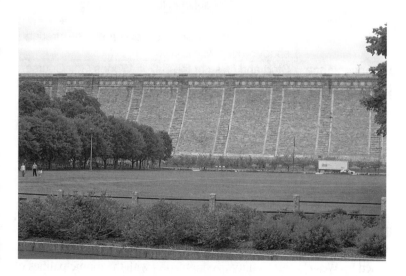

Kensico Dam Plaza

From the plaza, head north and west along the adjacent street, Broadway. Pass the school and continue on to the Valhalla shops. At the Cleveland Street pedestrian crossing go left across the parkway to the Metro North station.

Trains here are not as frequent as at North White Plains and south of there. However, there is an excellent place to wait for trains here. Valhalla Crossing restaurant and bar is one of the most charming eating and drinking establishments you will find anywhere. The environment is cozy and the food good. Enjoy your time here!

Colonial Greenway

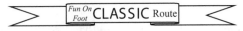

Distance	12.3 miles loop (Route WC8)
Comfort	Roughly two miles are on good street sidewalks, and the remainder of the route is on earth pedestrian trails of varying quality. The trails are mostly well defined and well used, but there are a few rough stretches and some moderate grades. Expect to pass other pedestrians on most parts of the route. Not suitable for inline skating.
Attractions	An interesting route through a variety of environments, including several stretches through shady woods with considerable wildlife.
Convenience	Start and finish at the Saxon Woods Golf Course on Mamaroneck Road, off the Hutchinson River Parkway at Exit 22. There is free parking here. You can also get to this route from the Mamaroneck Metro North New Haven Line station.
Destination	The Saxon Woods Golf Club is an excellent destination because it has a great casual pub/restaurant, the Saxon Grill, for winding down after this quite challenging route.

The Colonial Greenway is quite remarkable, being a long loop through a variety of parkland settings. It was cleverly put together and is maintained by Westchester County in conjunction with the municipalities of New Rochelle, Eastchester, Larchmont, Mamaroneck, and Scarsdale.

It includes trails through Saxon Woods County Park, Nature Study Woods County Park, and Twin Lakes County Park, plus the Leather-stocking Trail and part of the Hutchinson River Parkway Trail.

This route, on the east side of south Westchester County, is mostly good underfoot but may have you hiking rather than running at a few points. There are few interruptions from road crossings. You can start the loop at many different places, and choose to go either clockwise or counterclockwise around it. There are also some variations that involve doing less than the entire 12.3-mile outer loop.

We chose to feature the entire loop, going clockwise around it. We suggest starting at the Saxon Woods Golf Course in Scarsdale, for reasons of convenience and a good destination for winding down at the end. Assuming you are driving, this location is easily reached off the Hutchinson River Parkway at Exit 22. There is free parking, plus all the other facilities of a public golf course, including a public restaurant and bar.

VARIATION

If you are tied to public transit, an alternative starting point is the Mamaroneck Metro North station. From the station, go south (towards the rear of the train from New York City) to Mamaroneck Avenue. There are restaurants to the left here. Go to the right, (under the tracks if you arrived on a train from NYC). Cross the little creek and cross Mamaroneck Avenue to its south side. When the main road swings to the right, keep going straight up along Old White Plains Road. Cross Interstate 95 on the narrow sidewalk of the street bridge. After the bridge, there is no sidewalk and you need to walk on the edge of the road for about 200 yards to where the Leatherstock-ing Trail intersects the road. Since there can be considerable traffic, this can be quite dangerous. For that reason we are reluctant to recommend this option.

Exit the golf club, cross Mamaroneck Road, and note the Colonial Greenway map sign. These signs, strategically located along the route, are extremely helpful in advising exactly where you are and distances to various points ahead. Another helpful thing about this trail is the blazing. Sometimes there is a sheet-metal blaze with a circle of white stars on a blue diamond background. Other times the blaze is painted,

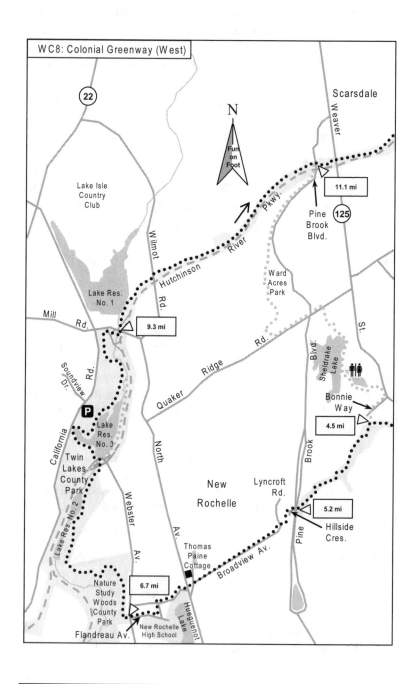

WC8: Colonial Greenway (West)

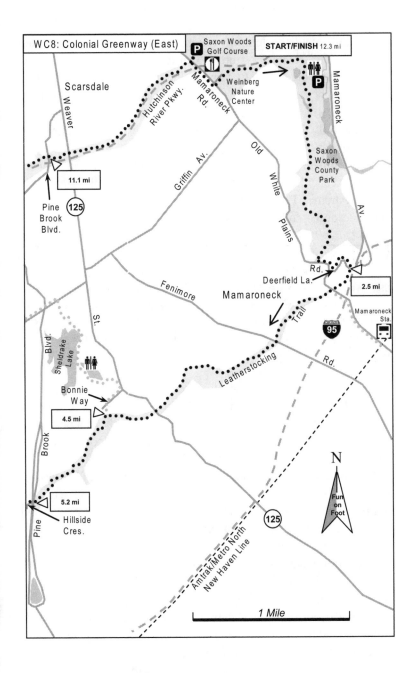

WC8: Colonial Greenway (East)

Saxon Woods Golf Course

START/FINISH 12.3 mi

Scarsdale

Weaver

Hutchinson River Pkwy.

Mamaroneck Rd.

Weinberg Nature Center

Griffin Av.

Old

White Plains

Saxon Woods County Park

Mamaroneck

Av.

11.1 mi

Pine Brook Blvd.

125

Rd.

Deerfield La.

2.5 mi

Mamaroneck Sta.

Fenimore

Mamaroneck

Trail

95

Rd.

St.

Blvd.

Sheldrake Lake

Leatherstocking

Bonnie Way

4.5 mi

N

Brook

Fun on Foot

5.2 mi

Hillside Cres.

Pine

125

Amtrak/Metro North New Haven Line

1 Mile

in which case it comprises a white star (or a white smudge) on a blue diamond.

Go left across the highway ramp, then over the parkway, and continue to the Weinberg Nature Center entrance. Cross Mamaroneck Road and enter the Nature Center. Follow the paved road to where it turns hard right near the building. Go straight ahead on the trail with the blaze. Follow the trail through the reserve—it can be a bit confusing so watch carefully for the blazes. Exit at a little gate and sign announcing the start of Saxon Woods County Park.

The trail here and most of the way through Saxon Woods County Park is excellent—a shady, wide, earth trail with mild grades but nothing extreme. The trail leads to public restrooms, near a parking lot with street access to Mamaroneck Avenue.

VARIATION

Saxon Woods County Park is a good on-foot exercise place in its own right. There are connecting trails down both the west and east sides. While the Colonial Greenway only uses the west-side trail, you can do loops through the park using both trails. Park in the lot off Mamaroneck Avenue, just south of the Hutchison River Parkway, or at the Weinberg Nature Center.

Pass the restrooms on your left. Continue following the wide trail and the blazes southward down the park. In the southernmost corner of the park, conditions change quite dramatically, with the trail becoming narrow, rocky underfoot, and steep in parts. The trail is not always easy to follow either, so watch carefully for the blazes.

The trail exits Saxon Woods County Park on Old White Plains Road, at a Colonial Greenway map sign. Go left along the edge of the road to the first street left, Deerfield Lane. Follow this quiet street around and down to the trailhead of the Leatherstocking Trail.

This is generally an excellent trail, snaking through a reserve along a creek bed in what is otherwise a residential area. It extends for 2.6 miles. The major risk factor with this trail is that it is close to water and marshlands and can be unpleasant in times of heavy rainfall. Even if it is good underfoot, bugs can be a problem. However, it has a wealth of wildlife including many birds and small mammals. There are several street crossings, where a little care is needed.

> **VARIATION**
>
> At the 5.2-mile point of our route, after crossing Weaver Street, you come to a trail junction with a trail heading north to Sheldrake Lake Larchmont Reservoir and Ward Acres Park. This is the south end of the "middle leg" of the Colonial Greenway, which you can use to craft loops shorter than the 12.3 miles of the full outer loop. If you go north here, it is 2.7 miles to connect to the Hutchinson River Parkway Trail at Pine Brook Boulevard. If you then pick up our main trail to finish back at the Saxon Woods Golf Course, your total loop distance would be 8.4 miles.
>
> Similarly you can craft a loop of only the west lobe of the Colonial Greenway with a length of 9.3 miles.

At the end of the Leatherstocking Trail you emerge in the City of New Rochelle on the edge of Pine Brook Boulevard. Cross the street and follow Hillside Crescent on the other side. This street leads you uphill to its dead end. At the end, however, is a small grassy path through to Lyncroft Road. Continue straight ahead into Broadview Avenue. This is a particularly beautiful residential street, lined by classy homes all the way. Proceed down the hill (noting the Colonial Greenway blazes) to North Avenue, where you can see Huguenot Lake to the left and the Thomas Paine Cottage to the right. This is the start point of the Paine to Pain Classic Trail Half-Marathon, which was first run in 2008 and which goes around the Colonial Greenway.

Cross North Avenue at the light, and follow the blazes around the lake, the park, and New Rochelle High School to Flandreau Avenue. This street leads down to Webster Avenue, which you cross to enter the next park in our series—Nature Study Woods County Park.

This park has a wealth of trails through it and is a popular training place for runners from the nearby high school and Iona College. There is usually ample parking in Webster Avenue or nearby, if you need that for local loop running.

To keep to the Colonial Greenway, bear hard right after entering the park and eventually you will become comfortable finding the blazes among the many trails that crisscross this park. Note that from now on, the Colonial Greenway trails are designated as equestrian as well as pedestrian. However, anything with wheels is prohibited.

The trail leads into Twin Lakes County Park, another beautiful park with wide, well-kept trails. The white swans that inhabit the first lake impressed us. Continuing northward, the trail follows the Hutchinson River under the Hutchinson River Parkway and then crosses the river. You then climb up to the little trail bridge over the parkway ramp. Across this bridge is a trail intersection. Go left, following the blaze.

VARIATION

There is a nice trail loop around the upper lake in Twin Lakes County Park, and the aforementioned trail intersection defines the southern end of that loop. Use this loop to build a local exercise route here. There is parking off California Road, near Soundview Drive, or run up and back from Nature Study Woods County Park.

The trail on the west side of the lake is very pleasant, being well removed from the parkway traffic. It goes up to skirt the edge of California Road. The trail then becomes rougher underfoot, rocky, and less level. You come to a trail T-junction. Go left (unless you are looping back around the lake per the variation noted above).

You emerge on the edge of Mill Road, where you exit Twin Lakes County Park. From this point on you follow the trail along the edge of the Hutchinson River Parkway. Cross the two lanes of parkway ramps. Take the trail around under Mill Street and climb up to the trail bridge over the parkway ramps. Cross Wilmot Road and go left across the parkway ramp.

The trail from here to the end is less used and less pleasant than what went before, owing largely to the incessant noise from the adjacent parkway. It is also less well cared for—it can be overgrown in parts, so beware of poison ivy.

At Pine Brook Boulevard you are where the middle leg of the Colonial Greenway meets the Hutchinson River Parkway Trail. See our prior variation box for options you might consider here.

Cross Pine Brook Boulevard and continue on to cross Weaver Street. In our experience this is probably the worst maintained part of the trail. But we encourage you to push on…

The trail emerges on Mamaroneck Road, directly across from the Saxon Woods Golf Course where you started. You will now likely appreciate why we chose this finish point. Attached to the golf clubhouse is the Saxon Grill, an excellent casual bar and grill. After that quite challenging on-foot outing, you just might be like me and be more than ready for an ice-cold beverage. Wind down here before heading home.

Franklin D. Roosevelt State Park

Distance	Various (Route WC9)
Comfort	There are various trails, some along roads and some through wilderness. Expect to pass other pedestrians on most trails. Not suitable for inline skating.
Attractions	Many trails, all well away from significant vehicle traffic.
Convenience	You need to drive here. There is an exit from the Taconic State Parkway directly into the park. There is ample parking in the park.
Destination	Enjoy the park's recreational facilities, including the massive pool and extensive picnic areas.

Franklin D. Roosevelt State Park is in the north of Westchester County, immediately west of Yorktown Heights. It has some excellent trails. You can obtain a rudimentary trail map from the park office.

There are essentially three different types of trail:

- Use the edges of the paved vehicle roads. Traffic is light and speed is limited to 25 mph, with the latter carefully monitored by the park police. This is a popular choice with park visitors.
- There are some very good, wide, vehicle-free trails, including a closed section of road and the fire roads that constitute the Nature Trail.
- There are many smaller, less used paths through the woods.

There are some grades but nothing extreme. We have included on our map only the first two categories of trail, with segment mileages shown. Use this information to craft whatever loop works for you. If you are seeking company running here, contact the Taconic Road Runners Club.

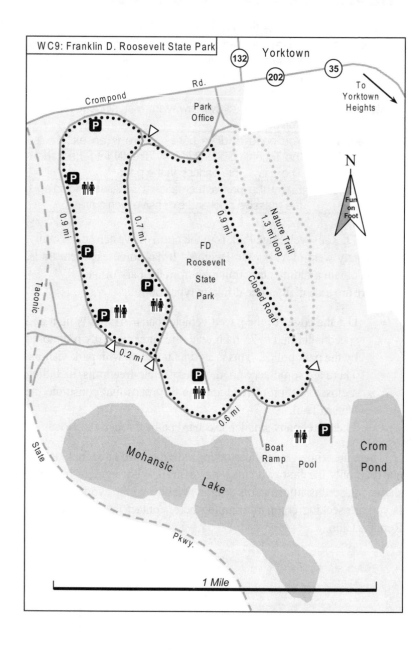

WC9: Franklin D. Roosevelt State Park

Yorktown

Crompond Rd.

Park Office

To Yorktown Heights

N

Fun on Foot

Taconic

State

0.9 mi

0.7 mi

0.9 mi

Nature Trail 1.3 mi loop

FD Roosevelt State Park

Closed Road

0.2 mi

0.6 mi

Mohansic Lake

Boat Ramp

Pool

Crom Pond

Pkwy.

1 Mile

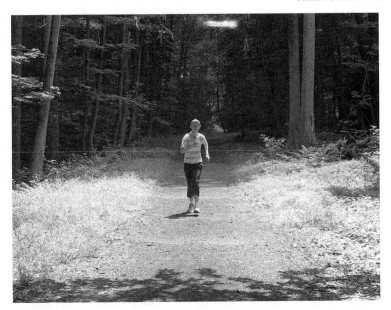

The Nature Trail in Franklin D. Roosevelt State Park

Other Routes

The **Briarcliff-Peekskill Trailway** is a pedestrian-only trail that runs from the Town of Ossining north to the **Blue Mountain Reservation** in Peekskill. The trail is built on land originally acquired in 1929 by the Westchester Parkway Commission for the construction of a parkway that was never completed. It passes through the Teatown Reservation and Croton Gorge County Park. There are extensive scenic trails in the Blue Mountain Reservation, which can be reached off Route 9 at Welcher Avenue.

There is some outstanding running in the region around the **New Croton Reservoir** south of Yorktown Heights. Among other options, you can connect to trails in the Kitchawan Preserve and from there to the North County Trailway. The Taconic Road Runners Club meets here every weekend. Check the club website for details.

The **North County Trailway** follows the right-of-way of the defunct Putnam Division of the New York Central Railroad from the Interstate 287 corridor in the south to the Putnam County Line in the north. Most of it involves a paved multiuse trail but some sections are along unpaved road shoulders. Route WC5 (Tarrytown Three-Trail Loop) used part of the Trailway south of Route 117. North of there the Trailway goes through Millwood, Kitchawan, and Yorktown Heights, to Baldwin Place and the county line. This is a great trail for local out-and-back running.

We have covered the **Old Croton Aqueduct Trail** from the Bronx up to the Rockwood Hall area of Rockefeller State Park Preserve. The trail continues north from there to the town center of Ossining (roughly three miles) and on to Croton Gorge Park at the base of the New Croton Dam (roughly five more miles). At Ossining you can reach the trail easily from the Metro North Hudson Line station. However, there are no other stations convenient to the trail. You can drive to Croton Gorge Park from Route 129 between Quaker Bridge and the New Croton Reservoir. If you are interested in exploring this part of the Old Croton Aqueduct Trail, we recommend you obtain a copy of the map and guide from the Friends of the Old Croton Aqueduct (available from the www. funonfoot.com website).

The **South County Trailway** is a paved multiuse trail following the Saw Mill River Parkway from Van Cortlandt Park in the south to the Interstate 287 corridor in the north. We covered the southernmost part in route BX8 (Van Cortlandt to Yonkers). The remainder of the Trailway is good for locals doing an out-and-back run. There is no convenient public transit linking different points on the Trailway so it is difficult to construct more interesting outings. Also there is considerable vehicle noise and pollution along the entire route from the parkway traffic and also Interstate 87 traffic in some parts.

Tibbetts Brook Park is in Yonkers between the Saw Mill River Parkway and the Old Croton Aqueduct, stretching from the Cross County Parkway in the north almost to the Bronx line in the south. There is excellent running here, including a pleasant two-mile loop. Route BX8 (Van Cortlandt to Yonkers) shows how to get to this park from either Van Cortlandt Park or the center of Yonkers.

Running Clubs

Sound Shore Runners and Multisport Club (www.soundshorerun.com)

This club has more than 275 members, from New Rochelle to Greenwich, Mamaroneck to White Plains. Club activities include regular morning, evening, and weekend group runs, weekly speed work sessions, trail runs, and social events. Anyone who seeks an active and healthy life is welcome to join. There are members who do fun runs, serious races, marathons, biathlons and triathlons, and no races at all. Young or old; slow or fast; long distance or short; new to fitness or veteran; singles, couples and families with children—everyone is welcome.

Email: Refer to website

Taconic Road Runners Club (www.runner.org)

The Taconic Road Runners Club, based in Northern Westchester County, is one of the premier racing clubs in the 40+ categories. However, most members run for fun. Running in club races is just as much a social event as it is a competition, and you do not need to be fast to join. Members run daily, with widely varying paces for all runners.

Email: Refer to "Important Information" page of website

Westchester Track Club (www.westchestertrack.org)

This club was founded in 1973 by Mike Barnow, who has coached it for almost 30 years. The Westchester Track Club is a two-tiered club for elite and recreational runners. The nationally registered track team (formerly Puma) consists of a multinational group of Olympic aspirants. The recreational group meets on Wednesday evenings (during the months of April through November) at White Plains High School for structured interval workouts. All are welcome to join.

Email: Refer to "Contact Us" page of website

9

Long Island

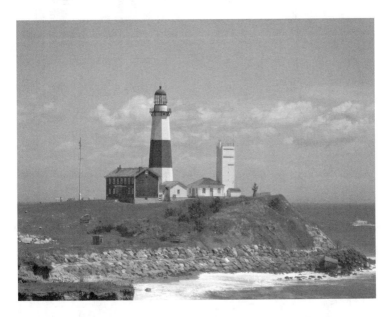

Long Island comprises the counties of Queens, Kings, Nassau, and Suffolk. The first two of these map to the New York City boroughs of Queens and Brooklyn, which we covered in earlier chapters. In this chapter we cover the rest of the island—Nassau and Suffolk counties.[1]

Long Island, which is over 100 miles long but only 23 miles wide at its widest point, is densely populated and crisscrossed with a busy road grid. Public transit is quite limited, with the automobile being the standard means of local travel. The Long Island Rail Road (LIRR) operates an extensive rail network, which is mainly a commuter service to New York City.

---

1   Chapter head photo: Montauk Point, Suffolk County.

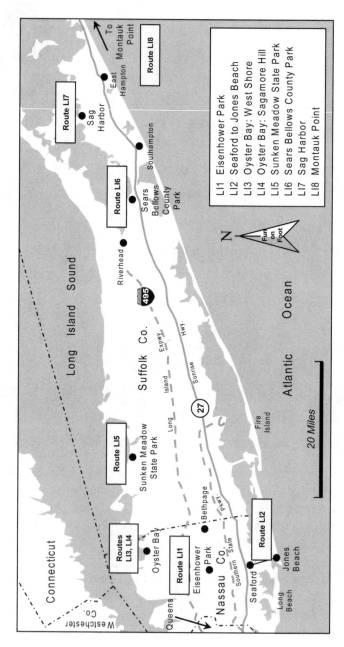

Long Island Routes

There are innumerable parks, many having paths suitable for outdoor exercise. For this book we decided to limit coverage to outdoor exercise places that are really outstanding and particularly popular with local runners and walkers. We are featuring eight routes, four in Nassau County and four in Suffolk County. Some of these routes can be reached on foot from LIRR stations.

Route	Distance
LI1 Eisenhower Park	Various
LI2 Seaford to Jones Beach	9.0 miles out/back
LI3 Oyster Bay: West Shore	5.6 miles out/back
LI4 Oyster Bay: Sagamore Hill	6.4 miles out/back
LI5 Sunken Meadow State Park	Various
LI6 Sears Bellows County Park	Various
LI7 Sag Harbor	5.7 miles loop
LI8 Montauk Point	Various

Eisenhower Park

Distance	Various (Route LI1)
Comfort	A popular park with excellent quality trails and many runners and walkers. Some paths are suitable for inline skating.
Attractions	Excellent running conditions, pleasant surroundings, measured marked trails.
Convenience	This park is central to Nassau County. You will probably drive here, although it is possible to get here on foot from the Westbury LIRR station (approximately one mile). The park is off Hempstead Turnpike (Route 24) between Meadowbrook Parkway and Wantagh State Parkway. Enter via Park Boulevard and park your vehicle in the first lot you come to on the left.
Destination	Enjoy the facilities of the park. If hungry or thirsty, there are some food and beverage establishments nearby on Hempstead Turnpike.

Eisenhower Park is a very attractive and popular park, with good facilities. There are ample restrooms, water fountains, an inline skating area, an aquatic center, tennis courts, sporting fields, and a pretty lake. There are several miles of paved running or walking trails. Furthermore, this park is home to the Long Island Road Runners Club, the predominant running club in this region. This park is also the site of the start and finish of the Long Island Marathon run in May.

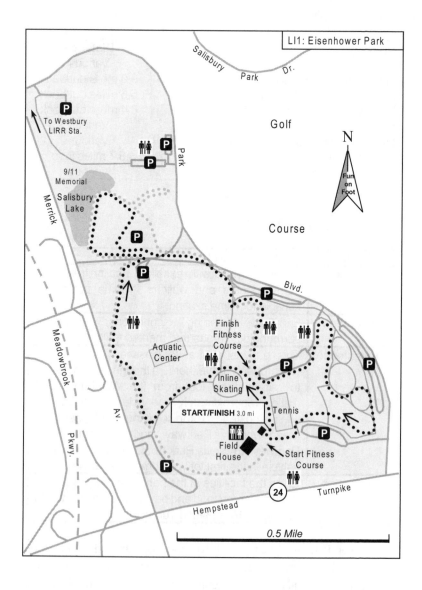

One feature of this park for the on-foot exerciser is the set of marked, measured running routes. There are three-, two-, and one-mile routes.

The marked routes start near the Field House, beyond the tennis courts next to Parking Field 2. Go to the little hut with the Long Island Road Runners Club sign. There are two main trails marked by colored arrows painted on the pavement—the red trail (3.0 miles) and the white trail (1.0 mile). There is also a 2.0-mile Fitness Course, with exercise stations along it. On our map we feature the red trail (black dots) and also show the fitness course (gray dots). Both of these routes go by the lake, where a tasteful 9/11 Memorial is located. You can vary these routes in many ways to your own liking.

If you seek food or beverages after your exercise, there are some restaurant/bars on Hempstead Turnpike.[2]

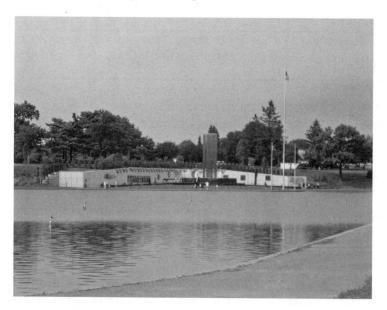

The 9/11 Memorial in Eisenhower Park

---

2   We thank Fred Haslett, President of the Long Island Road Runners Club, for introducing us to Eisenhower Park.

Seaford to Jones Beach

Distance	9.0 miles out and back (Route LI2)
Comfort	An out-and-back route on an excellent quality paved multiuse trail. Expect plenty of cyclists, inline skaters, and pedestrians. Excellent for inline skating.
Attractions	Nassau County's premier long paved multiuse trail, with plenty of fresh air and a beautiful and popular beach at the turnaround point.
Convenience	This route starts and finishes in Cedar Creek Park in Seaford, Nassau County. Drive to the park at Larch Street and Merrick Road, just east of Wantagh State Parkway. It is possible to get here on foot from the Wantagh LIRR station (approximately a half mile due north of the park).
Destination	If hungry or thirsty, there are restaurant/bars in walking distance of Cedar Creek Park on Merrick Road.

This is a very popular multiuse trail, used predominantly by cyclists but with a good number of inline skaters and runners as well. It links Seaford, a pleasant little center in the south of Nassau County off Route 27, to Jones Beach, one of Long Island's most popular swimming beaches.

Cedar Creek Park is a pleasant park adjacent to the center of Seaford. It has some paved trails of its own but, most significantly, it represents the northern end of the trail to Jones Beach following Wantagh State Parkway. There is ample parking in the park and you can easily walk or run here from Wantagh LIRR station.

Enter the park at Larch Street, off Merrick Road. Bear right around the entrance road. At the western extremity of the road loop there are restrooms and a trailhead to the Ellen Farrant Memorial Bikeway. From here it is 4.1 miles to the beach on the paved multiuse trail following Wantagh State Parkway.

The trail can be busy in the summer but is wide enough most of the way. You need to cross two bridges on sidewalks and the trail narrows at these points. The nearby road traffic definitely detracts from this route but, since it is close to the water, the air quality is not bad.

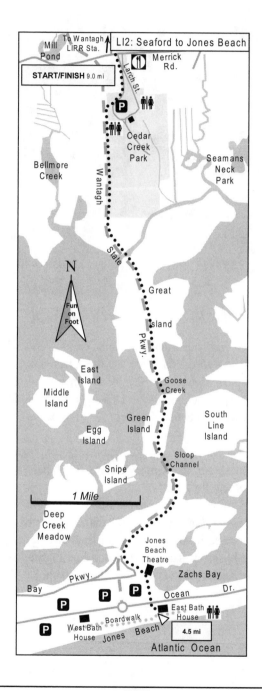

LI2: Seaford to Jones Beach

To Wantagh LIRR Sta.

Mill Pond

Merrick Rd.

START/FINISH 9.0 mi

Larch St.

Cedar Creek Park

Wantagh

Bellmore Creek

Seamans Neck Park

State

N

Fun on Foot

Great

Island

Pkwy.

East Island

Middle Island

Goose Creek

Egg Island

Green Island

South Line Island

Snipe Island

Sloop Channel

1 Mile

Deep Creek Meadow

Jones Beach Theatre

Zachs Bay

Pkwy.

Bay

P   P   P

Ocean   Dr.

East Bath House

P

Boardwalk

West Bath House   Jones Beach

4.5 mi

Atlantic Ocean

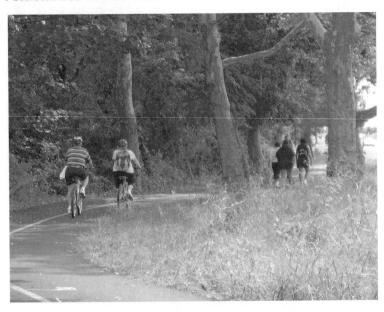

The Seaford to Jones Beach Trail

At the beach end, you emerge in a bike parking area where you can lock bikes. Across to the east you see the Jones Beach Theatre. Go across the car park towards the theatre and then south near the water of Zachs Bay. Approaching Ocean Drive you find a pedestrian tunnel under that highway. The tunnel brings you out near the East Bathhouse of Jones Beach.

Here you can exercise on the boardwalk, buy snacks, and use restrooms. There is an excellent swimming beach here, if you have the time and equipment for that.

Return to Seaford on the trail you used to get here. You might find the return trip easier than the outbound, thanks to a tailwind.

Back at the park, if you are ready for food or a beverage, there are some good establishments on Merritt Road near Fir Street. The popular (and quite spectacular) East Bay Diner is a good choice.

Oyster Bay: West Shore

Distance	5.6 miles out and back (Route LI3)
Comfort	An out-and-back route on a well used unpaved running trail with no vehicle crossings. Not suitable for inline skating.
Attractions	A beautiful trail along the shore of Oyster Bay. No interruptions from vehicle traffic.
Convenience	Start and finish in the center of Oyster Bay, near the LIRR station and Theodore Roosevelt Memorial Park. There is ample parking around here or you can travel here by the LIRR. Driving from the Long Island Expressway, take Route 106 north from Exit 41.
Destination	Oyster Bay is a pleasant town with all facilities. If hungry or thirsty, there are several restaurant/bars in the town center.

Oyster Bay is an attractive little town off Long Island Sound in the north of Nassau County. It is historically significant as the home of Theodore Roosevelt from 1886 until his death in 1919. This is the first of two Oyster Bay routes we chose to feature.

On the west side of Oyster Bay there is a beautiful trail following the shore and West Shore Road 2.8 miles to Bayville.

Start in Theodore Roosevelt Memorial Park, on the shore side of town near the LIRR station. Head west following the rail tracks. Find West End Avenue and follow it to Beekman Beach. At the west end of the parking lot there is a path to the trail along West Shore Road. This is a well used unpaved running path, between the road and the shore. The scenery along the edge of Oyster Bay is spectacular.

You come to the Bayville drawbridge. Cross the bridge and continue to the T-junction at Bayville Avenue. This is our nominal turnaround point. There is a pleasant village here, with services and a nice beach, but we suggest you simply retrace your steps back to Oyster Bay.

VARIATION

You can add on a loop to extend your return leg by about 3.6 miles. It goes through pleasant residential neighborhoods but involves considerable travel on road edges. Go left at Bayville Avenue, then left into Bayville Road, left into Factory Pond Road, and left into Cleft Road, which returns you to West Shore Road.

On getting back to Oyster Bay town center, there are several suitable placees for a drink or meal. We liked Canterbury Ales Oyster Bar and Grill in Audrey Avenue near the station.

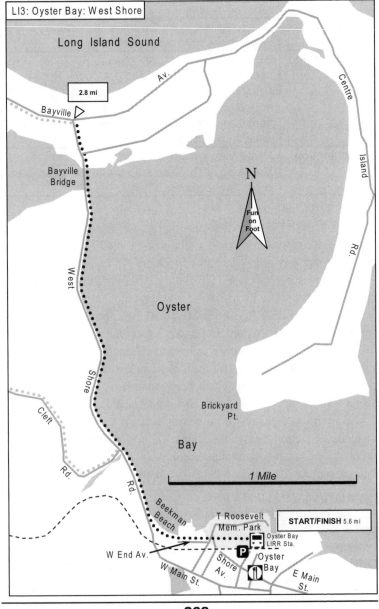

Oyster Bay: Sagamore Hill

Distance	6.4 miles out and back (Route LI4)
Comfort	An out-and-back route mostly on the edges of trafficked streets, with sidewalks the exception rather than the rule. Vehicle traffic is nearby but it is unlikely to be either heavy or fast. Avoid darkness hours. Expect to encounter a few other pedestrians but no crowds. Not suitable for inline skating.
Attractions	The main attraction is the Sagamore Hill National Historic Site, including the former home of Theodore Roosevelt.
Convenience	Start and finish in the center of Oyster Bay, near the LIRR station and Theodore Roosevelt Memorial Park. There is ample parking around here or you can travel here by the LIRR. Driving from the Long Island Expressway, take Route 106 north from Exit 41.
Destination	Oyster Bay is an attractive town with all facilities. If hungry or thirsty, there are several restaurant/bars in the town center.

This is our second Oyster Bay route. In this route we mix exercise and history by traveling on foot from Oyster Bay town center to the historic home of Theodore Roosevelt at Sagamore Hill. This was his home from 1886 until his death in 1919. If your main interest is in exercising, this is a great running or walking route with history as a sideline. If your main interest is in seeing the historic site, there is no better way to get to and from there.[3]

Start by the LIRR station near Theodore Roosevelt Memorial Park. Head east along Shore Avenue to South Street (Route 106). Continue straight ahead into East Main Street. East Main Street changes name to Cove Road. While there is no sidewalk here, there is a good, wide shoulder that is acceptable to most local runners.

At the intersection with Cove Neck Road, go left along that road. There is no sidewalk until Gracewood Court, but traffic is usually light and sedate. When the sidewalk starts, follow it to Sagamore Hill Road

---

[3]   Our motivation to explore this route stemmed from a web posting by Mike Polansky.

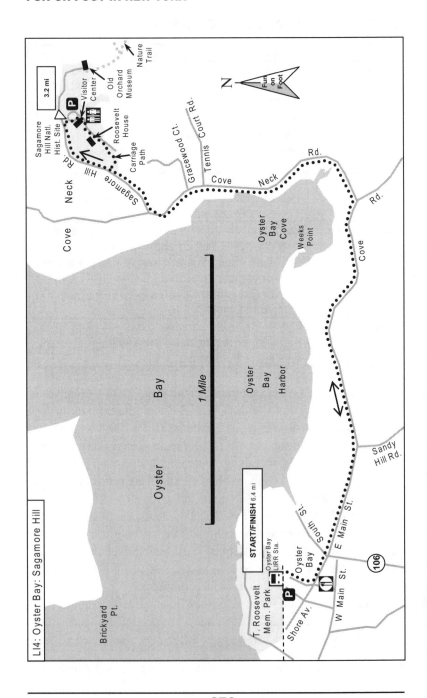

LI4: Oyster Bay: Sagamore Hill

3.2 mi

Sagamore Hill Natl. Hist. Site

Visitor Center

Old Orchard Museum

Nature Trail

Roosevelt House

Carriage Path

Neck Cove Rd.

Sagamore Hill Rd.

Gracewood Ct.

Tennis Court Rd.

Cove Neck Rd.

Oyster Bay Cove

Weeks Point

Cove Rd.

Oyster Bay

Oyster Bay Harbor

Oyster Bay

1 Mile

Brickyard Pt.

T. Roosevelt Mem. Park

Oyster Bay LIRR Sta.

START/FINISH 6.4 mi

Shore Av.

South St.

E Main St.

W Main St.

Sandy Hill Rd.

106

N Fun on Foot

and then along that road to the entrance to the Sagamore Hill National Historic Site. The entrance road takes you to the visitor center where there are restrooms and displays.

VARIATION

As you enter the Historic Site the road to the left leads to the Old Orchard Museum where there are exhibits and the park offices. Behind the museum is a trailhead for the Nature Trail, a loop of roughly one half mile through the forest to the east. From the nature trail you can get to a small beach on Cold Spring Harbor.

Go right around the visitor center and pass the Theodore Roosevelt house, bearing left on the paved trail. Near the end of the paved trail, there is an unpaved carriage road through the woods. It takes you back to Sagamore Hill Road. Retrace your steps to Oyster Bay and enjoy the hospitality of a local establishment there.

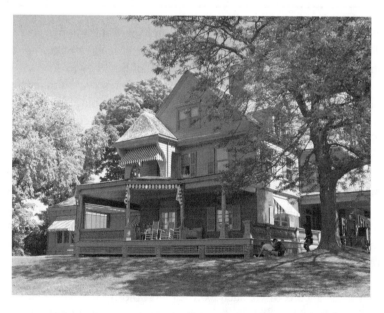

Theodore Roosevelt House, Sagamore Hill

Sunken Meadow State Park

Distance	Various (Route LI5)
Comfort	A popular beach and park with a boardwalk plus a network of cross-country trails. The latter are well used and well maintained unpaved trails, with some grades. Expect plenty of other pedestrians around. Not suitable for inline skating.
Attractions	Excellent running conditions, on well maintained earth trails without any concerns about vehicles. Plenty of greenery and wildlife.
Convenience	This park is at the north end of Sunken Meadow Parkway, which can be accessed off Exit 53 of the Long Island Expressway. There is ample parking in the park but a fee is charged seasonally.
Destination	Enjoy the facilities of the park, including its beautiful beach and picnic areas. There are snack outlets in season but no convenient restaurants or bars.

We now move east into Suffolk County for four routes in this county. The first place that warrants attention is Sunken Meadow State Park on the shore of Long Island Sound in the Town of Smithtown.

Sunken Meadow is a very pleasant recreation preserve with a popular beach. Furthermore, it is a particularly important place for runners because it hosts Long Island's most popular cross-country course. The vast majority of Nassau and Suffolk school students aspiring to a running future find themselves here at some stage.

There are regular cross-country courses for 5K, 10K, three-mile, and five-mile races. The 5K course is shown on the map. It weaves through a forested part of the park following a somewhat contorted route. It is mostly in the shade and has a sinter surface that is easy on the feet. For most of the route the grades are modest but the course has one renowned steep hill section known locally as Cardiac Hill. Overall it is considered one of the toughest 5K courses in the region. The longer distance courses, such as five miles, mostly use the same part of the park, with a slightly different route and with an additional loop extending into the section of the park closer to the Sunken Meadow Parkway entrance road.

There are innumerable trails in this park so you can easily craft your own route of whatever distance you wish. There is a pleasant boardwalk along the beachfront, which you can include in your route. There is a variety of wildlife in different ecological environments throughout the park.

When you have finished your exercise, you can buy a soda and a snack at one of the concession outlets and enjoy them on the beach.

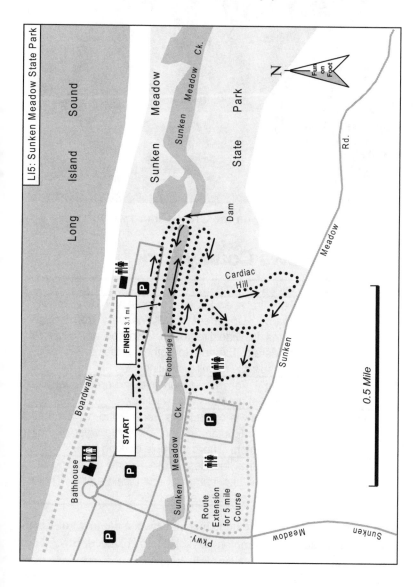

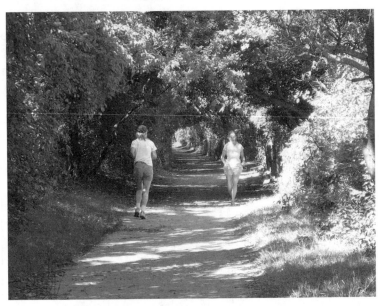

The Mousehole on the Cross-Country Course

Sears Bellows County Park

Distance	Various (Route LI6)
Comfort	Park trails and roads without vehicles, mostly shady. Underfoot conditions vary from rough paths to wide fire roads. Grades are slight to moderate. Expect a few other pedestrians around. Not suitable for inline skating.
Attractions	Escape from civilization into wilderness terrain. Plenty of greenery and wildlife.
Convenience	This park is off Bellows Pond Road, which runs between Routes 24 and 27 a little west of their intersection. There is ample parking here.
Destination	Enjoy the facilities of the park, including its beautiful lake, camping, and picnic areas. There are no food or beverage outlets.

This next Suffolk County route is inland, between the town of Riverhead and the hamlet of Hampton Bays, south of Flanders Bay. Sears Bellows Park has some excellent trail running in a forested environment.

You get to this park off Route 24 east of Riverhead. Bellows Pond Road heads off south of Route 24, about a mile west of the Route 27 junction. Go down this road to the park entrance on the right. There is a sizeable parking lot between the entrance and Bellows Pond. Campsites are also available. With good swimming in the pond in the summer, this is a popular camping destination.[4]

This park has hiking trails, dirt roads, and horse trails. Pedestrians are not supposed to use the latter, but the first two can be used for hiking or trail running as you choose. A rudimentary trail map is available from the office. We do not have accurate mileages for this route so can only give rough approximations.

The main hiking trails are blazed as follows:

- **Blue Trail:** This trail starts near the parking area and goes around Bellows Pond (roughly one mile). On the far side of the pond, the main branch of the blue-blazed trail heads off westward to Sears Pond.
- **Yellow Trail:** This trail goes around Sears Pond near the west edge of the park.
- **White Trail:** This trail is part of the Paumanok Path, which stretches 125 miles from Rocky Point to Montauk and cuts through the northwest corner of Sears Bellows Park.

We feature a loop that involves following the blue trail out to Sears Pond and returning via a road. This roughly 3.5-mile loop gives you a good introduction to the park, providing you all the information you need to maybe do something else next time.

Go either way around Bellows Pond to about the halfway mark, where there is a trail junction with another blue-blazed trail. That trail heads off directly away from Bellows Pond. Follow this blue-blazed trail about a half mile, crossing three horse trails and passing Division Pond on your right, to an intersection with a dirt road.

Cross the road and continue on the trail which is now both blue-blazed and white-blazed. The trail crosses another dirt road and winds almost a mile to a new trail intersection where the white-blazed trail goes to the left and a yellow-blazed trail goes to the right. There is a sign "To Sears Pond" pointing to the right. This trail takes you to a dirt road, where you go left to get to the edge of Sears Pond.

---

4   This route was recommended to us by Bob Beattie.

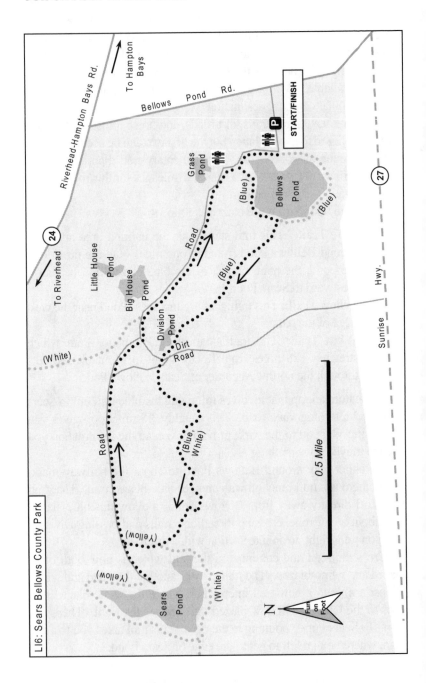

LI6: Sears Bellows County Park

VARIATION

At the sign you can alternatively go left and circumnavigate Sears Pond, getting you to the same point on the edge of the pond, but traveling about a half mile further. Part way around the pond, the white trail heads off to the west.

Sears Pond is quite pretty and popular with hikers in summer, but there are no facilities here.

To return to the park entrance, follow the dirt road (or retrace your steps on the hiking trail). Follow the road about a half-mile to a road branch and take the left branch. Continue to a T-intersection. Here you are close to Division Pond. Go left. Pass the trailhead for the white-blazed trail, which heads north to Red Creek Park on the north side of Route 24. Continue past Big House Pond on your left. Cross the horse trail and pass through the road gate to the main picnic and camping area. You come to restrooms on your left. The main parking area is a little further on.

There are no food or beverage outlets in the park so you need to drive a few minutes into either Hampton Bays or Riverhead for that.

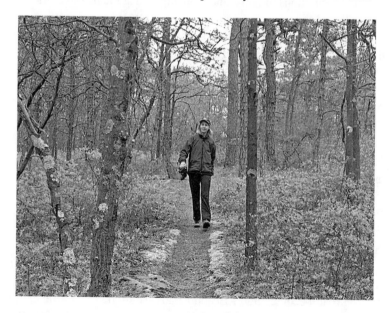

The Blue Trail in Sears Bellows Park

Sag Harbor

Distance	5.7 miles loop (Route LI7)
Comfort	This route uses street sidewalks and some road shoulders, the latter mostly being quite wide. There is moderate vehicle traffic in some parts. Expect to pass cyclists and some other pedestrians. Not recommended for inline skating.
Attractions	A quaint village environment plus some beautiful seaside scenery.
Convenience	Start and finish in the center of the village or at any other point on the loop.
Destination	The village center has many shops and some historic attractions. There are several restaurants and bars for a wind-down meal or beverage.

Sag Harbor is a fascinating historic village, very popular with tourists in summer. It is an old whaling town, first settled in 1707. The village center, with plenty of interesting shops, restaurants, and bars, is adjacent to the port. We happened to be in Sag Harbor for its 300th anniversary celebrations in 2007, and were amazed at the massive, friendly crowd there.

For the on-foot exerciser, there is an excellent 5.7-mile loop along the streets through the village center and around Sag Harbor Cove.

Start at the top end of Main Street at Route 114 near the wharf. Go south down Main Street on the sidewalk. Pass the whaling museum. At Brick Kiln Road go right and then right again into Noyack Road. The sidewalks cease to exist on this stretch and the pedestrian is forced to use the road shoulder. Turn right where Noyack Road and Stoney Hill Road meet. Continue to the intersection with Long Beach Road and go right again.

The next mile, along Long Beach, is particularly pleasant. Pedestrians can use a side road that services car parking, escaping the through traffic. The view of Noyack Bay is very scenic and the sunsets can be spectacular.

When the side road ends you are forced back to following the main road, which has wide shoulders with bike lanes on both sides.

The road becomes Short Beach Road. Continue to a traffic circle. Go right along South Ferry Road, Route 114. The shoulders are still nice and wide here.

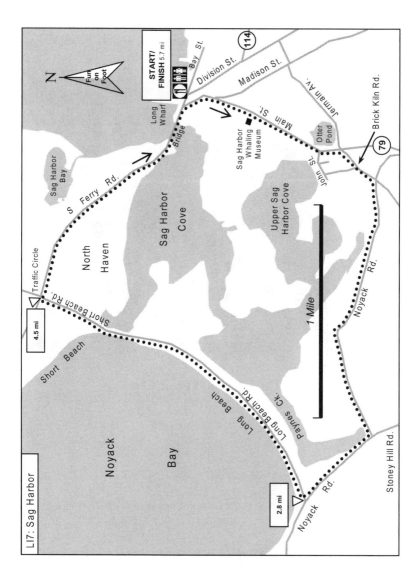

As you approach the bridge, a sidewalk starts on the right side of the road and leads onto the bridge ramp. Cross the bridge, enjoying the spectacular views of the sea and the village. This brings you back to the village center where this route started.

There are public restrooms near the wharf on Bay Street, past the old windmill (now a visitor center). There are several eating and drinking establishments around here. We like the Corner Bar at the top end of Main Street at Route 114.

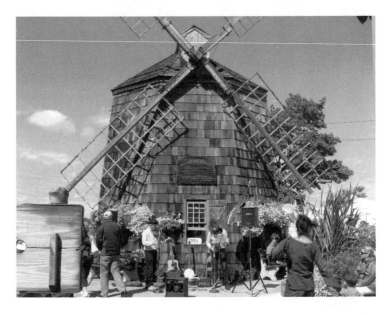

The Historic Mill Visitor Center

Montauk Point

Distance	Various (Route LI8)
Comfort	Unpaved pedestrian trails, with underfoot conditions varying from old roads to twisty hiking trails and a little scrambling over rocks. Expect to pass other pedestrians. Not suitable for inline skating.
Attractions	Some stunning coastal scenery, numerous points of historic interest, and considerable wildlife.
Convenience	Start and finish by the lighthouse at the tip of Montauk Point. To drive here follow Route 27 to its eastern end. There is ample pay parking here.
Destination	Tour the lighthouse and admire the spectacular views. There are restrooms and snacks here. For a more substantial food or beverage establishment drive back to Montauk center.

Montauk Point is the extreme easterly tip of Long Island. It is a truly spectacular place. It is a place that everyone must visit and, when here, we strongly recommend you take the opportunity to explore the area on foot and get some great exercise at the same time.[5]

We feature a loop of Montauk Point, including Camp Hero State Park. This route differs from our usual type of route, being unquestionably more a hiking trail than a running trail for much of its length. However, this loop is so special we just had to include it. We do not have accurate mileages for this loop, but would estimate it at five-to-six miles. It took us two hours to complete at a solid hiking pace.

Drive to Montauk Point and park in the pay lot near the lighthouse. There are restrooms, snacks, and information here.

Go down the path on the north side of the lighthouse to the water. Walk carefully on the rocks around the water below the lighthouse. This is not particularly dangerous, but it is definitely not a running activity either. You come to a trailhead. Note the white blazes that identify the Paumanok Path. These blazes are very important in successfully navigating this route. The Paumanok Path is a 125-mile hiking route extending to Rocky Point. It endeavors to trace the path used by the indigenous people prior to European civilization here.

---

5   This route was recommended to us by Bob Beattie. For more details of hiking trails around here, see *Trail Guide to the South Fork* by Mike Bottini, The Southampton Press, 2003.

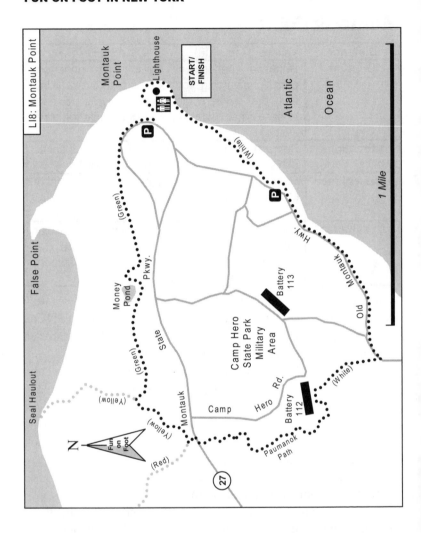

The trail initially twists uphill through stunted wilderness. It emerges at an ocean overlook near a radio tower. Follow any of the trails along the top of the bluff, to a small parking lot. The path then joins a gravel road. The conditions are excellent for running on this part of the route. Proceed to the stretch where there are numbered parking spaces for fishing licensees. Pass the road to the left to the Bluff Overlook. You come to a sign indicating Point Woods Trail and Paumanok Path West. The signs also make clear that the trails are for hikers only; no bikes, horses, or ATVs. Signs also warn of unexploded ordinance, so it might be a good idea not to stray far from the trails.

The Paumanok Path trail is initially earth with some grass and is excellent for trail running. Follow the white blazes and emerge at the Battery 112 site. The 16-inch guns that were housed here could fire up to 25 miles out to sea. Follow the earth road to the left. Keep following the blazes carefully as the trail becomes progressively rougher underfoot and harder to follow. Now you are in serious forest hiking terrain. It takes time to get to the highway because the trail twists so much. It took us over an hour to get from the lighthouse to the highway.

Cross the highway and go 100 yards to the right to the trailhead. There are signs and blazes here. Go in 50 yards to more explanatory signs. Follow the sign for the Seal Haulout Trail (yellow blaze) and the Money Pond Trail (green blaze). This is a good quality trail, suitable for trail running. Initially the blazes are all yellow. After roughly a half-mile you then come to a trail intersection clearly marked for the Money Pond Trail—take that and follow green blazes thereafter.

VARIATION

You can take a diversion here up to the shore and back on the yellow-blazed trail. There is a scenic view over Long Island Sound here and, with luck, you will see plenty of seals. This diversion adds roughly a mile to your route.

Skirt Money Pond on your left. This is where Captain Kidd is supposed to have buried his treasure. We encountered significant wildlife around here, including deer and a fox.

After a certain amount of trail weaving, climb a headland to emerge at an overlook of the water, close to the highway. When you reach the highway, you can see the lighthouse and the café.

After this trek, you might wish to tour the lighthouse and take in the scenery some more. If you want food or beverages, we suggest you drive back to Montauk center. We can personally recommend two fine establishments here—the Shagwong Tavern in Main Street and the Montauket. For the latter go up Edgemere Road to Tuthill Road to Fleming Road. It is an amazing place for a drink at sunset.

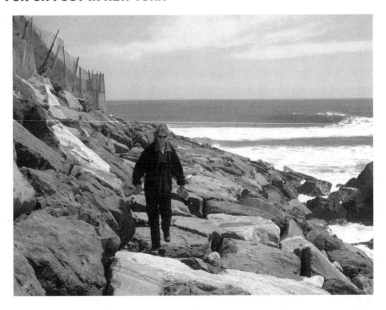

The Start of the Trail is Scenic but Rocky

Other Routes

Here are some other interesting routes we encountered in Nassau County.

The **Bethpage-Massapequa Bike Path** extends 6.5 miles from Bethpage State Park south to Route 27 in the Massapequa County Preserve, with a one-mile extension further south to Merrick Road. You can park in Bethpage State Park by the picnic area, at Route 27 (off Lake Shore Drive), or at Merrick Road (off Ocean Avenue). The path is of excellent quality but close to a busy road for part of the way. You can get to the trail from the Bethpage LIRR station by walking east on Powell Avenue or from the Massapequa LIRR station via a path from the station parking lot. There is a white-blazed hiking trail following the general course of the paved multiuse trail. The hiking trail extends north from Bethpage State Park to Cold Spring Harbor.

The City of **Long Beach** has a 2.2-mile boardwalk popular with local runners, joggers, walkers, and cyclists.

The **Muttontown Preserve** is south of Oyster Bay off Route 106. Alternatively you can start at the nature center off Route 25A, where you pick up a trail map. It has some pleasant trails with a variety of terrain and wildlife. They are mainly considered hiking trails but are suitable for cross-country running.

* * * *

Here are some other routes in Suffolk County.

In **Blydenburgh County Park** in Smithtown there is a trail loop of roughly four miles around New Mill Pond. The headquarters of the Long Island Greenbelt Trail Conference is also here; you can obtain maps of several interesting Long Island hiking trails from this organization.

Fire Island is a popular beach resort in the southwest of Suffolk County, accessible only by ferry. Traversing the long foreshore can be very pleasant, but do it early morning before the crowds hit the narrow paths.

The **Long Island Greenbelt Trail** is a 33-mile blazed trail linking Sunken Meadow State Park to Heckscher State Park near Islip on Great South Bay. Obtain more information and maps from www.hike-li.com or www.ligreenbelt.org.

There are several miles of trails in **Mashomack Preserve** on Shelter Island, north of Sag Harbor. Go north from Sag Harbor and cross by ferry. The park entrance is on the right off this main road.

We touched on the 125-mile **Paumanok Path** in two featured routes in this chapter. There are several other places where you might access segments of this trail. For more information refer to the www.hike-li.org website.

There is a fascinating little trail called the **Walking Dunes** in Hither Hills State Park, on the west side of Montauk. From Route 27, take Napeague Harbor Road north to its end. Here you find a one-mile self-guided trail with details of how the dunes migrate into the forest and eventually out again. It is not for running training but interesting nonetheless.

Running Clubs

Bellmore Striders (www.bellmorestriders.com)
A small club with members aged from 23 to 51 focused on training from 500 meters to marathons. The club meets three days per week year-round.
Email: bellmore-striders@juno.com

Bohemia Track Club (www.btc.org)
The Bohemia Track Club, on the south shore of Suffolk County, offers a variety of activities to both the recreational and competitive runner, covering track and field as well as road running. The club welcomes runners and joggers of all ages and abilities. The only requirement is that you be involved with running in some aspect and want to connect with others with the same interests. Members vary in age from the 20s to the 70s. The club meets on the third Wednesday of each month at the Bohemia Recreation Center in Bohemia.
Email: membership@btc.org

East End Road & Trail Runners Club (www.eerunner.org)
The club's mission is to promote running, develop races, and inform the community of runners. Races support health, fitness, and educational and environmental needs. See the website for forthcoming events.
Email: bob@eerunner.com

Greater Long Island Running Club (www.glirc.org)
The club's mission is to promote running and fitness on Long Island for people of all ages and levels of ability. There are monthly meetings, weekly track workouts (April-October), fun runs, a monthly magazine, support of charities (especially those related to running and fitness), triathlon and running clinics, and support of a club racing team.
Email: spolansky@aol.com

Long Beach Road Runners Club (www.lbrrc.org)
The club's primary goal is to promote the sport of running to all ages throughout the Long Beach community. It also welcomes runners from neighboring communities such as Lido Beach, Island Park, Oceanside, Atlantic Beach, and Point Lookout. In addition to promoting the City of Long Beach running events, the Long Beach Road Runners host three other events: New Years Day 5k, Lobsterfest 5K, and World Run Day.
Email: lbrrc@yahoo.com

Long Island Road Runners Club (www.lirrc.org)
LIRRC has been serving runners for thirty-two years with over 80 events yearly in scenic Eisenhower Park. The club features: spring and fall marathon tune-up races; quarter-, half- and one-mile summer series kids and youth fun runs; a 5K summer series; cross-country races; 4 x 2-mile relay; and BBQs.
Email: mail@lirrc.org

Massapequa Road Runners (www.massapequaroadrunners.org)
The Massapequa Road Runners club was established 27 years ago and operates out of Massapequa Park. The club meets every second Tuesday of the month and club members enjoy running locally and traveling out to other area events, plus many social activities. Their big family race of the season, which is well attended, is the Firecracker Race held on the July 4th weekend. It consists of a 5K or a combination "Lift 'n Run" which is unique to the area.
Email: massapequaroadrunners@yahoo.com

New Hyde Park Runners' Club (www.nhprunners.com)
The club has regular runs Tuesday through Sunday. Runs are from five to seven miles with longer runs of up to 23 miles for runners training for a marathon. There are pace groups for runners of all types. Several members are also triathletes. The club hosts the New Hyde Park five-mile race and one-mile fun run, on the first Sunday in June.
Email: bcshja@msn.com

Northport Running Club (www.nrcrun.org)
This club hosts the Great Cow Harbor 10K Race and conducts up to four weekly group runs for runners of varying paces.
Email: Refer to website

10

Upstate New York

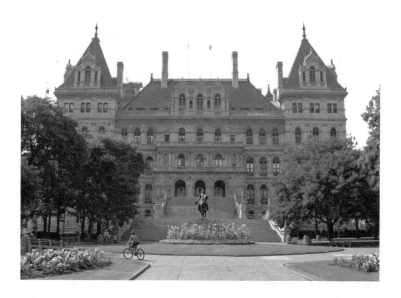

T his chapter covers centers in New York State outside of New York City, Westchester County, and Long Island, which were covered in prior chapters.[1]

Upstate New York has many cities and innumerable outdoor exercise trails. Our coverage in this book is, by necessity, extremely limited. In our available space, we opted to feature 11 routes that are close to major centers of the region, that we really enjoy, and that we consider worthy of note. If you happen to be visiting one of these centers, check out these routes. They are presented in order of distance from New York City.

---

1   Chapter head photo: The New York State Capitol in Albany.

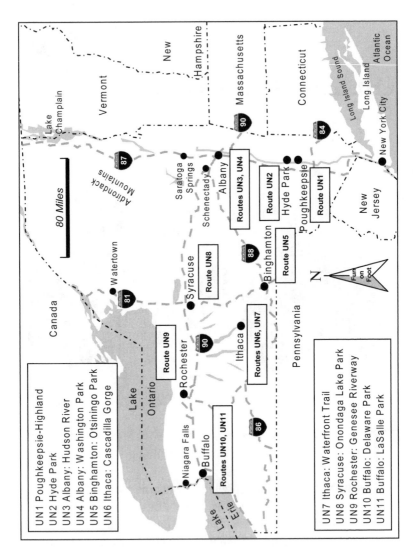

Upstate New York Routes

UN1 Poughkeepsie-Highland
UN2 Hyde Park
UN3 Albany: Hudson River
UN4 Albany: Washington Park
UN5 Binghamton: Otsiningo Park
UN6 Ithaca: Cascadilla Gorge

UN7 Ithaca: Waterfront Trail
UN8 Syracuse: Onondaga Lake Park
UN9 Rochester: Genesee Riverway
UN10 Buffalo: Delaware Park
UN11 Buffalo: LaSalle Park

Routes UN3, UN4
Route UN2
Route UN1
Route UN5
Route UN8
Route UN9
Routes UN6, UN7
Routes UN10, UN11

Route	Distance
UN1 Poughkeepsie-Highland	4.3 miles loop
UN2 Hyde Park	Various
UN3 Albany: Hudson River	2.6 miles loop
UN4 Albany: Washington Park	3.7 miles loop
UN5 Binghamton: Otsiningo Park	5.4 miles out/back
UN6 Ithaca: Cascadilla Gorge	1.4 miles out/back
UN7 Ithaca: Waterfront Trail	4.0 miles loop
UN8 Syracuse: Onondaga Lake Park	9.6 miles out/back
UN9 Rochester: Genesee Riverway	7.0 miles loop
UN10 Buffalo: Delaware Park	7.7 miles loop
UN11 Buffalo: LaSalle Park	4.1 miles loop

In the Other Routes section, we summarize some additional route ideas in a variety of places.

Poughkeepsie-Highland

Distance	4.3 miles loop (Route UN1)
Comfort	Paved surfaces throughout, with some grades. Roughly half the route is on sidewalks with vehicles nearby; the rest is on streets with very little traffic. There are virtually no vehicle cross-traffic interruptions. Inline skating is possible, but be prepared for some significant grades and rough parts.
Attractions	An excellent running training route. Enjoy the fresh air and scenic views from the Hudson Bridge.
Convenience	Start and finish at the Amtrak station close to downtown Poughkeepsie. There is parking here.
Destination	Poughkeepsie's Waterfront District, with restaurants, bars, and a pleasant park.

Poughkeepsie, where New York State ratified the U.S. Constitution in 1788, is a major population and business center in the Hudson corridor between New York City and Albany. This city is on the Hudson River's east bank, roughly 100 miles from New York City. Long being home to a major IBM development campus, Poughkeepsie is also an important travel destination.

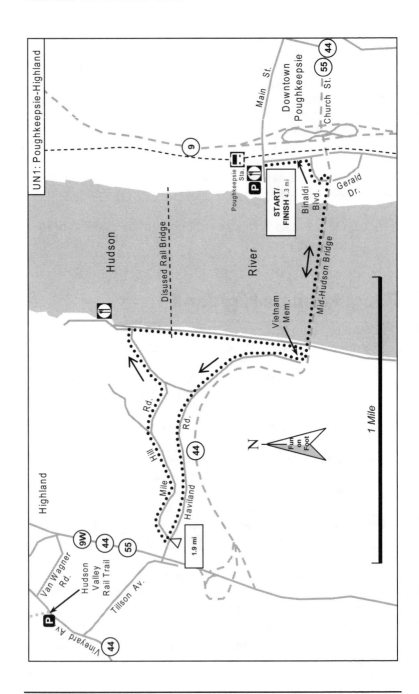

We found one excellent on-foot exercise route, starting and finishing in downtown Poughkeepsie. This route crosses the Hudson, an opportunity pedestrians rarely get. The scenery is spectacular, there are virtually no vehicle traffic encounters, and there are hills that make for a good workout if you are a runner in training.

Start at Main Street and Binaldi Boulevard, near the Poughkeepsie Amtrak station. The station is a few blocks down Main Street from the city heart at Market Street and is easily accessed on foot despite the generally invasive highway and rail tracks. There is ample parking near the station.

Follow Binaldi Boulevard south and turn right into Gerald Drive and a modern residential area. As you approach the Mid-Hudson Bridge that towers above, you come to a paved ramp heading up to the left. Follow this ramp to the bridge's northern walkway.

Cross the walkway of this impressive suspension bridge. While the zooming traffic is not far away, the bridge superstructure separates the traffic and pedestrians somewhat. The spectacular views compensate for any discomfort from the traffic noise.

At the west end of the bridge, pass the descending staircase and bear right into the peaceful parking area of the Johnson Iorio memorial to

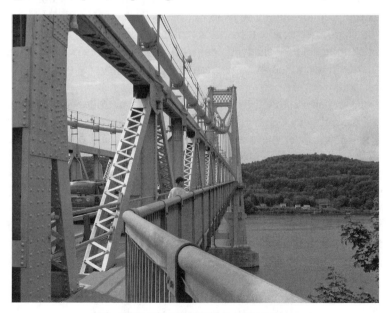

The Mid-Hudson Bridge Walkway

local Vietnam War veterans. A paved road, Haviland Road, starts here. Follow that road up the hill. There is little traffic so, if you do not mind the uphill grade, it is an excellent exercise route. The road takes you up to eventually meet the busy highway variously called Route 9W, Route 44, or Route 55, on the outskirts of the town of Highland. There is a gas station on the corner.

VARIATION

You can continue on foot from here towards the college town of New Paltz. There is a popular, paved rail trail called the Hudson Valley Rail Trail from the center of Highland to the Town of Lloyd and beyond. It currently goes 2.5 miles from Vineyard Avenue to Tony Williams Park. You can get to the start of the trail from the end of Haviland Road via Tillson Avenue and Vineyard Avenue. There is a project planned to extend the rail trail east to Haviland Road (targeted for completion in 2009). There is also a longer-range plan to extend the trail west to the New Paltz line, making it 7.5 miles long in total. (Thanks to Ray Constantino for this information.)

Just before the Route 9W intersection, there is a road heading off Haviland Road to the right called Mile Hill Road. Take this road downhill, following the signs to Mariner's Restaurant on the Hudson. This is another excellent road for running or walking. There is very little traffic, and the shady, green, ferny environment is very relaxing. Proceed down to the riverfront, arriving just downstream of Mariner's Restaurant.

From here, follow the paved road downstream following the river and the rail tracks. Expect little traffic here, since it is not a through road. Pass under the old high-level rail bridge and onward to the highway suspension bridge. Close to that bridge, you need to find an unmarked paved drive between two houses that leads up to the steps to the bridge level. Climb the steps to the bridge walkway, near the Vietnam memorial.

Retrace your steps to our start point at Main Street and Binaldi Boulevard. This is an excellent place to end an exercise outing. There is a nice park for winding-down and some good food and beverage establishments here in the Waterfront District. After such an enthralling and tiring run, Nola and I enormously enjoyed the hospitality of Mahoney's Irish Pub and Restaurant in Dooley Square.

> **VARIATION**
>
> There are plans to open up the old Poughkeepsie-Highland Railroad Bridge across the Hudson as a pedestrian walkway and bicycle path. When this spectacular *Walkway Over the Hudson* is complete it will add many exciting new options for running or walking routes in the Poughkeepsie-Highland region. Look to building a loop using that bridge and the route described here. For latest status check www.walkway.org.

Hyde Park

Distance	Various (Route UN2)
Comfort	These trails are generally wide, well maintained pedestrian trails, mostly earth but paved in some parts. Expect to meet other pedestrians on all trails. Not suitable for inline skating.
Attractions	There is something for everyone here. There are fascinating historic sites, beautiful scenery, escape from crowds and vehicles, and some excellent trail running for the athlete in training.
Convenience	You can start and finish the Hyde Park trails at many different points and craft your own outings. There are some loop trails, with convenient parking. There are also interesting ways to link trails together. Consider operating as a team and leaving a vehicle in advance at your planned finish point.
Destination	Choose your own destination, including various historic sites or restaurant/bars.

Hyde Park is a quiet little town on the Hudson's east bank, roughly six miles upstream of Poughkeepsie. Despite the quietness, it is a major tourist destination and has tremendous appeal for anyone with the Fun-on-Foot mentality.

Hyde Park is the center of three majestic historic estates, all now managed as National Historic Monuments—the home of Franklin D. Roosevelt, the Eleanor Roosevelt Historic Site, and the Vanderbilt Mansion. All of these estates have pleasant carriage roads and foot trails. The local community has built upon those resources by linking all three sites together by connectors to give the *Hyde Park Trail*. This trail is clearly marked with white circular markers bearing a blue symbol.

You can run the entire Hyde Park Trail but, depending on your desired distance, you might want to operate as a team and leave a vehicle at the finish point. For shorter distances, there are several excellent trail loops through beautiful outdoor settings with historic sites nearby.

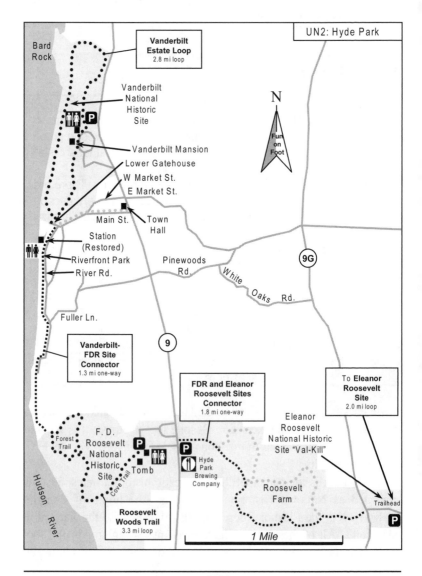

We therefore cover the Hyde Park trails as a set of optional segments, highlighting the combinations that make most sense.

Vanderbilt Estate Loop (2.8-mile loop; optional 0.6-mile connection to town center): The Vanderbilt estate has an excellent running or walking loop, which combines non-trafficked roads and off-road trails. It offers scenic views and some hills for those seeking a workout. You can drive to the Vanderbilt National Historic site and park there, to do the 2.8-mile loop. Alternatively, you can easily get to the loop from the town center, should you be based there. The latter option makes for a four-mile roundtrip. From the town center go down Main Street and continue down West Market Street/River Road to near the riverbank, where you see the old railroad station on the left. Bear right and enter the gates of the Vanderbilt Estate. Find the trail marker at the trail junction near the Lower Gatehouse.

Vanderbilt-FDR Site Connector (1.3 miles one way): You can get from the Vanderbilt Estate Lower Gatehouse entrance to the F. D. Roosevelt National Historic Site trail system on-foot. Go past the restored railroad station and through Riverfront Park. Then follow the edge of River Road, parallel to the river. River Road is narrow and a

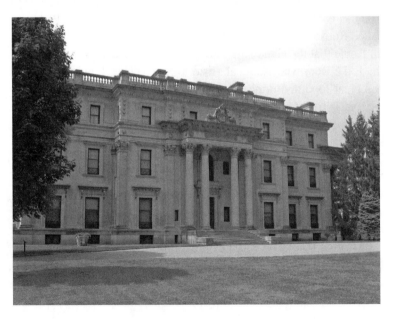

The Vanderbilt Mansion

little hilly. It has no sidewalk, but traffic is light. There are no river views after Riverfront Park, but the houses hugging the riverfront are quite impressive. The road ends at a paved turnaround circle. Look for the white trailhead marker near the fire hydrant. This trail connects you to the Forest Trail of the Roosevelt Woods trail system on the F. D. Roosevelt National Historic Site. This trail segment can be muddy underfoot, depending on season.

Roosevelt Woods Trail (3.3 miles loop): The F. D. Roosevelt National Historic Site has its own trail system called Roosevelt Woods. The trails are well marked and well maintained. There are a few trail choices but the best one (which is also marked as the Hyde Park Trail) involves taking the Cove Trail from the trailhead near the rose garden (where F. D. Roosevelt is interred) towards the river. Then take the Forest Trail off to the right before reaching the water. The Forest Trail is a 2.2-mile loop, giving a total round-trip length of 3.3 miles from the rose garden. To do this, drive and park in the historic site parking lot, off Route 9 south of Hyde Park. Alternatively, you can use the site connector described above to get to this site on-foot from the Vanderbilt Mansion or the town center.

FDR and Eleanor Roosevelt Sites Connector (1.8 miles one way): You can connect between these sites via a part of the Hyde Park Trail called Roosevelt Farm Lane Trail. The key access point is a trailhead on Route 9 at the Hyde Park Brewing Company, across the road from the F. D. Roosevelt National Historic Site. (The Brewing Company has great food and drinks, so is also a good place to finish up a big day out.) To get here from the F. D. Roosevelt National Historic Site, simply head east from the visitor center, bearing right to the secondary site access road (not the main entrance, which is a little further north). There is a good trail through the woods from the Route 9 trailhead to the Eleanor Roosevelt site, marked with the usual white round markers. The going is generally very good, through a pleasant forested area. There are several unblazed side trails, but they deserve caution since one can become lost.

Eleanor Roosevelt Site (2.0-mile loop): From the parking lot of the Eleanor Roosevelt National Historic Site (also known as Val-Kill), you are offered choices of a two-mile and a one-mile loop. Both trails are hilly in parts.

There are many ways to slice and tie these trail segments to make a nice on-foot outing. Here are three loop suggestions:

- Starting and ending in the town center, connect to the Vanderbilt Estate Loop and return to the town center (approximately four miles);
- Starting and ending at the Hyde Park Brewing Company, cross the road to the F. D. Roosevelt site and do the loop of the Roosevelt Woods Forest Trail. Enjoy the hospitality of the Brewery afterwards (approximately four miles);
- Starting and ending at the Hyde Park Brewery, connect to the Eleanor Roosevelt site and do the two-mile loop there. Enjoy the hospitality of the Brewery afterwards (approximately six miles).

Albany: Hudson River

Distance	2.6 miles loop (Route UN3)
Comfort	Roughly half a mile is on a paved pedestrian trail along the riverbank. The remainder is on street sidewalks along the river or in the downtown area. Expect plenty of other pedestrians around. Not recommended for inline skating.
Attractions	The fresh air and scenic views of the Hudson River, plus a tour of the city's core.
Convenience	Start and finish in the heart of downtown Albany at State Street and Pearl Street.
Destination	On weekdays there are plenty of things to see and do around the city center and there are several excellent restaurant/bars in or near Pearl Street. The business district largely shuts down on weekends.

Albany, the capital of New York State since 1797, is an attractive, pleasant, history-rich city. The city core is clean and well policed, with many good restaurants. People tend to have a laid-back attitude.

The city's overall crime rate is higher than we like to see—12.98 violent crimes per 1,000 inhabitants in 2006, roughly double the rate of New York City. However, in the parts of Albany that we cover, we found nothing that would concern the average runner or walker.

We feature two excellent Albany routes, both close to downtown. Both routes start and finish at State Street and Pearl Street, the intersection we would consider the center of Albany's heart. You might, of course, wish to adapt these routes to start or end elsewhere.

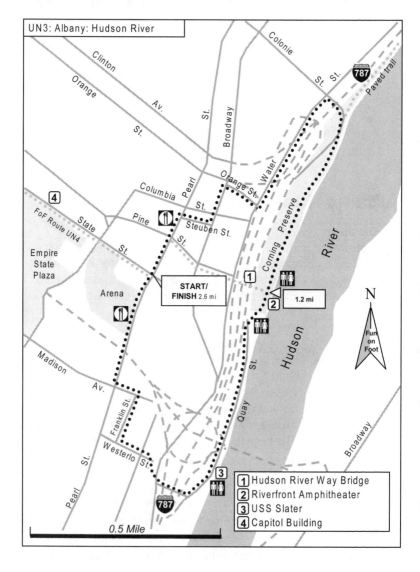

UN3: Albany: Hudson River

START/FINISH 2.6 mi

1.2 mi

N
Fun on Foot

1 Hudson River Way Bridge
2 Riverfront Amphitheater
3 USS Slater
4 Capitol Building

0.5 Mile

Albany has a lovely riverfront park, extending through the Corning Preserve, which is a venue for local events and for lunchtime exercise for downtown workers. This park has a good, paved multiuse trail.

The easiest way to the park is via the Hudson River Way pedestrian bridge over Interstate 787, east from the intersection of Pine Street and Broadway. However, there are other access points both upstream and downstream. We describe a 2.6-mile loop route using two such access points, but variations that use the Hudson River Way Bridge will be obvious.

Start at the intersection of State Street and Pearl Street. Go north up Pearl Street, past two streets off to the right, to the pleasant little lane to the right called Steuben Street. Steuben Street takes you to Broadway. Go left, cross Columbia Street, and go one block to Orange Street. Orange Street takes you to Water Street, which runs along the edge of Interstate 787. Follow the sidewalk of Water Street under the highway ramps to the intersection with Colonie Street, where you can take the sidewalk under the highway and into the riverfront park.

You find the paved multiuse trail here. It is a very pleasant trail along the riverbank, with plenty of shady trees. Take the trail to the right, downstream.

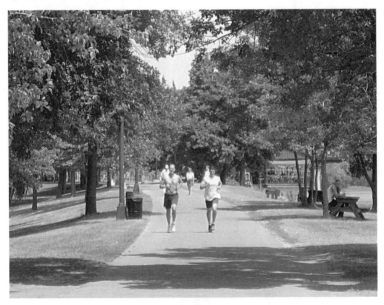

The Albany Riverfront Trail

VARIATION

The paved trail continues roughly four miles upstream from here. Go out and back on this excellent riverside trail.

The downstream trail leads you to the Riverfront Amphitheater, and the river end of the Hudson River Way bridge. Continue beyond the amphitheater to the end of the multiuse trail. There are restrooms here, and you can continue on the paved path along the edge of Quay Street. Go under the highway bridge that crosses the river. Shortly after the bridge you come to the *USS Slater*, the only World War II destroyer that remains afloat in the U.S.A. today.

After the *USS Slater*, follow the first street under the highway back into Albany proper. This is the Pastures district of Albany. It is not the city's nicest part, so you probably will not want to spend excess time here. To get back to central downtown, bear right into Westerlo Street. Follow it two short blocks to the pleasant little lane called Franklin Street. Go right into this lane and follow it to its end at Madison Avenue. Go left into Madison Avenue and then right into Pearl Street.

Proceed past the arena to our start point at State Street. If you feel the need for a food or beverage break, there are several good establishments around this part of Pearl Street.

Albany: Washington Park

Distance	3.7 miles loop (Route UN4)
Comfort	Roughly one mile of this route is on excellent trails in a very pleasant park. Roughly a half-mile is through the paved Empire State Plaza. The remainder is on street sidewalks. Expect plenty of other pedestrians around throughout. Not suitable for inline skating.
Attractions	Enjoy the escape from crowds and vehicles in Albany's most pleasant park. See some of Albany's major points of interest including the State Capitol, Empire State Plaza, and the Vietnam Memorial.
Convenience	Start and finish in the heart of downtown Albany at State Street and Pearl Street.
Destination	On weekdays there are plenty of things to see and do around the city center and there are several excellent restaurant/bars in or near Pearl Street. The business district largely shuts down on weekends.

This route involves a loop from downtown, through Albany's loveliest park and through Empire State Plaza, which houses the city's main convention center. If you want to start or finish at the convention center, the route adjustments will be obvious.

From State and Pearl Streets, go up State Street to the New York State Capitol. This majestic building, which is built entirely of masonry and incorporates a mixture of architectural styles, took 30 years to complete from its beginning in 1865 (see photo at chapter head).

Skirt the State Capitol bearing left and continue up State Street across Lark Street to Willett Street, where Washington Park starts on your left. Enter the park and work your way up its east side.

Washington Park has one somewhat annoying aspect—the traffic that zooms through on some roads on its east side. However, do not be overly concerned since natural beauty takes over in the west side of the park.

Follow the in-park road to the intersecting street heading left to the Park Playhouse. Expect little vehicle traffic now. Proceed towards the Playhouse and bear right to lovely Washington Park Lake. Circumnavigate this lake, without using the footbridge. There is an

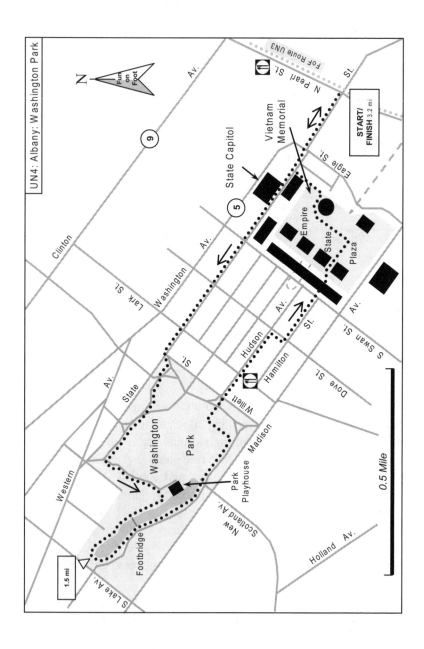

UN4: Albany: Washington Park

excellent, wide gravel trail up the east side. After the tip of the lake, come down the west side on a nice grass and earth trail.

Pass the Playhouse across the lake and come to the park's New Scotland Avenue entrance. You now have a variety of path choices to get back to Willett Street at the Hudson Avenue park entrance.

From the park entrance, go down Hudson Avenue to Lark Street. There is a nice collection of bars and restaurants here. Nola and I did this route on a very hot summer day and we greatly enjoyed the comfort of a Lark Street sports bar for a break at this point.

Continue south down Hudson Street and switch at some point one block west to Hamilton Street. Hamilton Street leads you directly into Empire State Plaza.

Take the stairs down and then up to the plaza level. Continue south between the high-rise towers into the main plaza. Your experience here will depend on the current weather and the scheduled events. At most times you can easily negotiate the plaza, but major crowd events happen here. Pass by the fountains and pools, and form your own opinion on whether this 1960s-70s architecture extravaganza is an enormous community asset or a concrete blight on an otherwise charming city décor.

Head towards the unmistakable egg structure, the performing arts auditorium.

Go around the egg and down the stairs towards downtown. These stairs lead you past the New York Vietnam Memorial and the courtyard honor roll in tribute to those New Yorkers killed or missing in action during that war.

Continue out of Empire State Plaza into State Street, and head to the right back to this route's start point.

Binghamton: Otsiningo Park

Distance	5.4 miles out and back (Route UN5)
Comfort	The entire route is on paved multiuse or pedestrian trails, excellent underfoot. There are no interruptions from vehicle cross-traffic. Expect plenty of other pedestrians around throughout. Suitable for inline skating.
Attractions	A very pleasant escape in an attractive and popular park. An excellent trail, equally good for strolling or athletic training.
Convenience	Start and finish at Otsiningo Park North at Howell Drive off Route 11. There is parking here.
Destination	There are fast food outlets, family restaurants, and stores near the finish.

Binghamton is at the confluence of the Susquehanna and Chenango Rivers, near the southern boundary of central New York State in Broome County. The tri-city Greater Binghamton region comprises Binghamton, Port Dickinson, and Johnson City. The region hosts Binghamton University, part of the SUNY system. The crime rate in Binghamton is a moderate 4.52 violent crimes per 1,000 inhabitants in 2006.

This region is highly automobile dependent. However, we found one outstanding on-foot trail along a three-mile stretch of the west bank of the Chenango River, north of central Binghamton. This is Otsiningo Park.

To use this trail you need to drive and park at either the north or south end and do an out-and-back run or walk. We chose to work from the north end.

Go up Route 11 to Howell Drive, which is immediately north of where Interstate 81 crosses over Route 11. There is a large supermarket here and several other shops, including some food outlets. Go past the shops to the Otsiningo Park North soccer fields and parking lot. There are restrooms here.

Go through the parking area to its south end where a wide paved trail starts. This trail is popular with walkers, runners, inline skaters, and cyclists. The river is nearby, making it quite pleasant. Interstate 81 is also nearby but not near enough to be a major problem.

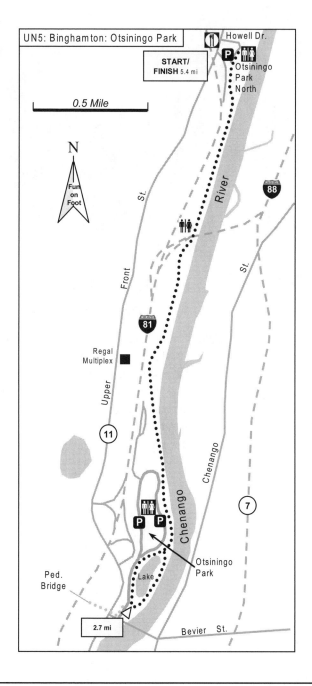

UN5: Binghamton: Otsiningo Park

Howell Dr.

START/ FINISH 5.4 mi

Otsiningo Park North

0.5 Mile

N

Fun on Foot

River

St.

88

Front

St.

81

Regal Multiplex

Upper

11

Chenango

Chenango

7

Otsiningo Park

Ped. Bridge

Lake

2.7 mi

Bevier   St.

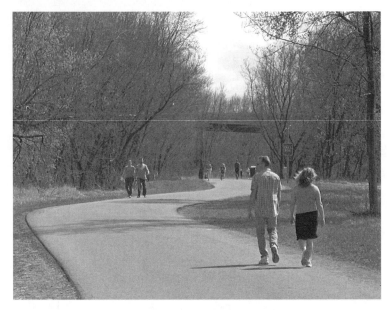

The Otsiningo Park Trail

Go under the Interstate-88 river flyover bridges. Continue down to the main part of Otsiningo Park. This park, accessed by road from Bevier Street, is a very popular place, with picnic areas, playgrounds, and sporting fields. There are restrooms here. At the south end of the park, at Bevier Street, there is a pedestrian overpass across Interstate 81 to residential areas and the Ely Park Municipal Golf Course.

We suggest you continue down to the park's lake, do a loop around it, and retrace your steps to Otsiningo Park North.

Ithaca: Cascadilla Gorge

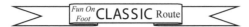

Distance	1.4 miles out and back (Route UN6)
Comfort	The gorge trail is 0.5 mile each way. It is paved but steep, and includes many steps. It can be wet and slippery in spots. The connection to the city center is 0.2 mile on good street sidewalks. Expect plenty of other pedestrians around throughout. Not suitable for inline skating.
Attractions	Spectacular scenery, including several cascades and waterfalls. A very practical connection between the city center and Cornell University campus.
Convenience	Start and finish at the corner of E Seneca Street and N Aurora Street in the city center close to downtown hotels. Alternatively, start and finish on the edge of campus, at the College Avenue Stone Arch Bridge.
Destination	There are restaurants, bars, and stores near both ends.

Ithaca, the home of Cornell University, is a lovely city at the bottom end of Cayuga Lake. It is an easygoing city, with a very modest crime rate (2.08 violent crimes per 1,000 inhabitants in 2006). We found three irresistible on-foot exercise places here: Cascadilla Gorge, the Cornell campus, and the Waterfront Trail.

Cascadilla Gorge, which connects downtown Ithaca with the Cornell campus, is a must-do route. It is probably the most spectacularly scenic route in this book. It is equally appealing in either direction. If you are downtown, do an out-and-back trip up to the campus, optionally exploring the campus or taking a lunch break there. If you are located on campus, come downtown, do your shopping or have a lunch break here, and return to campus. For our description, we assume the former. (You could also do the trail in just one direction, catching a bus the other way.) The trail is closed between sunset and dawn.

Start downtown at the intersection of E Seneca Street and N Aurora Street. Go north up N Aurora Street to Court Street. Go right one block and pick up the trail heading east along Cascadilla Creek. The trail

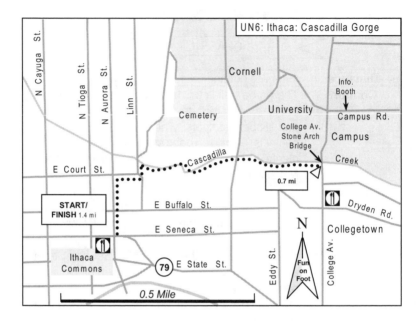

follows the edge of the creek up a gorge through a series of spectacular cascades and waterfalls. It is a substantial climb—over 400 feet. Some people run the trail but, if you do so, be very careful since the rocky path and steps are wet in places and can be slippery.

At the top of the gorge, the trail emerges at the south end of the College Avenue Stone Arch Bridge. For some ideas on exploring the campus, see the next section of this chapter. If you want a food or beverage break, go down College Avenue a block south from the bridge into the Collegetown area where there are shops and various food and beverage joints.

If you are at the downtown end of the trail and want a food or beverage break, there are many restaurant and bar choices around the Ithaca Commons, which is the shopping area south and west of our nominal start point. Nola and I like the Moosewood Restaurant in E Seneca Street near N Cayuga Street. Moosewood is a popular vegetarian restaurant, made famous by its series of cookbooks as much as its served food. We can also recommend Kilpatrick's Publick House in N Tioga Street near E Seneca Street.

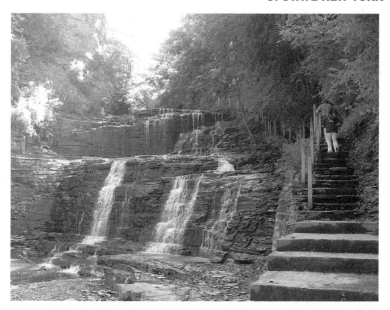

Cascadilla Gorge

Ithaca: Cornell Campus

The Cornell campus is particularly attractive—spacious, with many trees. It is also graced with the Cornell Plantations, an outstanding display of plant life covering a large area. The campus is an excellent place for outdoor exercise. There are limitless possible routes you might take through the campus and the Plantations. We saw no point in recommending any particular route, so instead chose to simply give a little information to help you get started on your own explorations.

Furthermore, we do not provide a map since you will be best served by picking up a free campus map at any of the information booths on campus.

The campus has two main sections, Central Campus and North Campus, on the south and north sides respectively of Fall Creek.

If you arrived at the campus via Route UN6 (Cascadilla Gorge) you will be at the College Avenue Stone Arch Bridge, on the southern edge of Central Campus. To start from here, cross Cascadilla Creek to its north side, via the Stone Arch Bridge. Then follow College Avenue north to

Campus Road and turn right. This takes you past an information booth where you can pick up a campus map to guide the rest of your visit.

The most attractive on-foot exercise places on campus are along Fall Creek at the northern edge of Central Campus. We particularly recommend doing a loop of Beebe Lake (roughly one mile). This involves crossing the creek via the Triphammer Footbridge at the west end of the lake and the Sackett Footbridge at the east end.

East of Beebe Lake are the Cornell Plantations, with various trails through them. On the west side of Judd Falls Road is the Botanic Garden area. You do a loop of the paved road around the treed area that encircles the rhododendron collection. This circuit takes you past the Plantations information office, and offers access to restrooms.

On the east side of Judd Falls Road is the Mundy Wildflower Garden area. There is a loop trail of roughly one mile through here. However, the trail is narrow and unpaved, so maybe not a wise choice for a road runner in training. If that is not a concern and you like wilderness and plant life, proceed through the Wildflower Garden and, optionally, continue on further east, across Caldwell Road, to the F. R. Newman Arboretum.

If you are a runner and will be spending a semester or more at Cornell, you should join one of the local running groups. A classic group is the High Noon Athletic Club, which meets at noon on campus every weekday for 5-to-10-mile runs in the surrounding area. For pointers to this and other groups, check out the website of the Finger Lakes Runners Club (www.fingerlakesrunners.org).

If you are visiting Ithaca and Cornell on a day trip and want a food or beverage break before returning downtown via the Cascadilla Gorge, go back to the Stone Arch Bridge, and south a block down College Avenue to the Collegetown shopping area.

Ithaca: Waterfront Trail

Distance	4.0 miles loop (Route UN7)
Comfort	The Waterfront Trail is a 2.2-mile paved trail loop through parkland. The connection to the city center is 0.9 mile each way on street sidewalks. Expect plenty of other pedestrians around throughout. The Waterfront Trail is good for inline skating, but the street connection is questionable.
Attractions	Pleasant scenery and excellent underfoot conditions on the Waterfront Trail.
Convenience	Start and finish at the corner of E Seneca Street and N Cayuga Street in the city center, close to downtown hotels.
Destination	There are restaurants, bars, and stores downtown near the finish point.

Start downtown at the intersection of E Seneca Street and N Cayuga Street, adjacent to the Ithaca Commons, the pedestrian mall where much of the life of Ithaca is centered.

Go up N Cayuga Street to W Buffalo Street and then head west on the sidewalk. Pass Washington Park. Cross the two branches of Cayuga Inlet. From here on you have trail signs to follow. Pick up the multiuse trail north, signposted as the Waterfront Trail. This trail is very popular on nice summer days with exercisers and families. The trail does a 2.2-mile loop up Cayuga Inlet and through Cass Park, almost as far north as the marina. There are restrooms in Cass Park.

At the north end of the loop you pass an entrance into Alan H. Treman State Marine Park. You can enter that park but there are no defined trails there.

Continue on the trail back to the bridge at W Buffalo Street and retrace your footsteps back to downtown. There are many choices of restaurant or bar just east of our nominal end point, should you feel like a wind-down snack or beverage.

There are plans for future extensions of the Ithaca Waterfront Trail system on the eastern side of Cayuga Inlet. Planning is underway for a trail from W Buffalo Street up to the Farmers Market, and also a trail from the Farmers Market, around the Newman Municipal Golf Course, up to Stewart Park. To check current status of these plans, visit the website www.cayugawaterfronttrail.com. Note that you can also connect from the Farmers Market to the Cascadilla Gorge Trail and Cornell University via the pleasant streets along the Cascadilla Creek outlet canal.

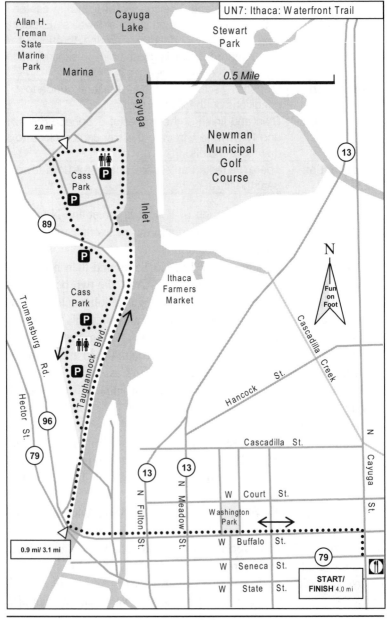

Syracuse: Onondaga Lake Park

Distance	9.6 miles out and back (Route UN8)
Comfort	There is a paved multiuse trail the entire route with no motor vehicle crossings. Expect plenty of other pedestrians around throughout. Good for inline skating.
Attractions	A very pleasant lakeside environment.
Convenience	Start and finish at the park's visitor center off Route 370. There is parking here or you can catch the Route 48 bus to Cypress Street and Route 57.
Destination	Explore the Salt Museum or enjoy the park facilities. There are limited food outlets nearby.

Syracuse is a city with a population around 150,000, at the crossroads of the major Interstates 90 and 81. It is home to Syracuse University and a mixture of industries. It is effectively the metropolis of the scenic Finger Lakes region of New York State. Unfortunately, the natural beauty of Syracuse has been compromised by indiscriminate highway construction in years past. Being a highly vehicle dependent city, pedestrian trails and even sidewalks have not been high on the city's agenda until recently.

However, there is one outstanding outdoor exercise location, quite close to downtown. Onondaga Lake Park is a beautiful and popular outdoor recreation location, which is being continually improved. Anyone visiting Syracuse must make a serious effort to spend some quality time on foot here.

Statistically, Syracuse has a relatively high crime rate—10.66 violent crimes per 1,000 inhabitants in 2006. However, we have seen nothing to particularly alarm us in the Onondaga Lake Park vicinity.

Onondaga Lake Park was a very popular location around the turn of the century, with amusement parks, promenades, and entertainment venues. In the mid-20th century it, like so many other similar places, became neglected. Highway Interstate 690 demolished the best parts of the west side, and the lake became polluted. In recent years, recovery has blossomed, with recognition of this area as an Onondaga County Park.

Today, Onondaga Lake Park is visited by an enormous number of runners, walkers, and cyclists every day. There are ample vehicle-free trails for everyone. The main trail is particularly good for inline skaters.

You virtually need to drive to the park (or catch a Route 48 bus from downtown or Liverpool; see www.centro.org for details). There is no practical way to get here on foot except on Sunday mornings in summer when the authorities close the parkway from the Carousel Center (the shopping center at the lake's southeast end) to the park for cyclists and on-footers.

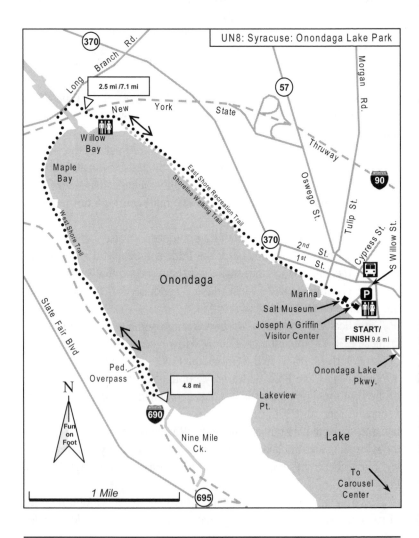

Start at the Joseph A. Griffin Visitor Center, at the lake end of S Willow Street. There are two paved trails up the lake from here to its northwest end. The East Shore Recreation Trail is heavily used by cyclists and inline skaters in summer. Snow is cleared in winter. The Shoreline Walking Trail is closer to the shore and popular with pedestrians in summer. Choose whichever works best for you.

Go 2.25 miles to Willow Bay, where there is a picnic area and year-round restrooms. In summer, there is a tram service back to the visitor center. The tram runs hourly; more frequently on weekends. If you only want to do 4.5 miles, this is a good turnaround point.

To continue around the lake, follow the trail on to the one-lane truss bridge across the outlet channel. This leads to the West Shore Trail down to Nine Mile Creek and the area where the amusement parks once were. If you turn around at the end and backtrack to the visitor center, the total distance is 9.6 miles. You also have an option of diverting onto the unpaved Lakeland Nature Trail off the West Shore Trail.

On returning to the visitor center, there are limited food outlets nearby. You also have the opportunity to explore the Salt Museum.

There is a plan to extend the trail the full 12 miles around the lake. This will be excellent when completed, but that may be some time off.

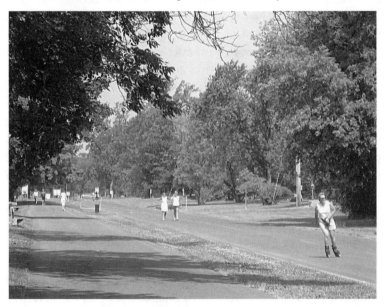

The Onondaga Lake Park Trail

Rochester: Genesee Riverway

Distance	7.0 miles loop (Route UN9)
Comfort	The entire route is on dedicated pedestrian or multiuse trails, mostly paved but unpaved in parts. Expect plenty of other pedestrians around throughout. Restrooms are scarce. Not suitable for inline skating overall.
Attractions	A pleasant riverside trail loop with several optional bridge crossings that allow you to create your own distance variants. A very practical connection between downtown and the University of Rochester campus.
Convenience	Start and finish at the corner of E Main Street and South Avenue in downtown Rochester, close to the Riverside Convention Center and downtown hotels.
Destination	There are many restaurants and bars near the finish point.

Rochester, with a population of almost 200,000, is New York State's third-largest city. Located conveniently close to and between the Lake Ontario shore and the New York State Thruway, it is a thriving center of industry and home to the University of Rochester.

For the on-foot exerciser, Rochester's appeal lies in its location at the crossroads of the Genesee River and the Erie Canal, both of which provide corridors for on-foot trails.

Most significantly, there is an excellent trail system along the Genesee River—the Genesee Riverway Trail. We chose to feature the section from downtown south to Genesee Valley Park and back. It passes by the edge of the University of Rochester campus. There are trails on both sides of the river and several bridges so you can pick your own distance and create your own loop.

Rochester statistically has a relatively high crime rate—12.60 violent crimes per 1,000 inhabitants in 2006. Use due caution but do not let that figure keep you at home.

Our featured route starts at E Main Street and South Avenue, by the Riverside Convention Center. Go down the sidewalk of South Avenue to Court Street. Here you see the first sign for the Riverway Trail. Continue south to the trailhead. Follow the trail under Interstate

490 and on to the Ford Street bridge where you could cross the river if desired. We recommend continuing along the riverbank on the pleasant, paved trail to the University of Rochester.

VARIATION

You can cross the river at the University of Rochester footbridge and return downtown on the other side. The total distance traveled would be approximately five miles.

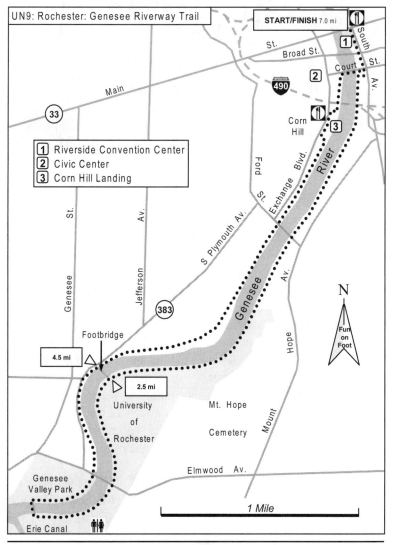

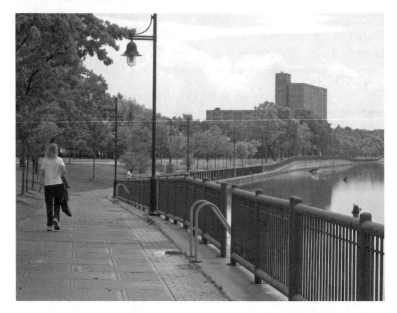

The East Bank Riverwalk Trail

Continue past the campus to the Elmwood Avenue Bridge. You can cross the river here too. Continue on to Genesee Valley Park, where there are picnic areas, sporting fields, and restrooms. Cross the river on the footbridge in this park.

Proceed north along the riverbank trail past the Elmwood Bridge and the University of Rochester footbridge. The trail then moves away from the river and passes through a quite secluded wooded area. It then joins a straight rail-trail, and the surroundings open up. The trail then reverts to the riverbank and leads into the Corn Hill area. You arrive at Corn Hill Landing, a popular area with a marina and shops. The buildings force you away from the riverbank. Across the road is Nathaniel's Pub, an excellent watering hole with a good pub-food menu.

Watch for the Riverwalk sign and go through the riverside buildings at this point. Follow the trail north under the Interstate-490 bridge. Continue on the trail to Court Street. Cross the river here and go back up South Avenue to our start point.

If you are ready for a food or beverage break, there are various pubs and restaurants around here. We can vouch for the Main Street Bar and Grill on E Main Street near the riverbank.

Buffalo: Delaware Park

Distance	7.7 miles loop (Route UN10)
Comfort	This route involves 2.9 miles on excellent park trails and 4.8 miles on reasonable street sidewalks connecting between the park and downtown. Expect plenty of other pedestrians around throughout. The 1.5-mile loop around the east lobe of Delaware Park is good for inline skating.
Attractions	A very pleasant Olmsted-designed park setting.
Convenience	Start and finish at the corner of Allen Street and Main Street, less than a mile from central downtown and the convention center. The start and finish point is convenient to several hotels.
Destination	There are several restaurants and bars near the finish, including the famous Anchor Bar. The Theodore Roosevelt Inaugural National Historic Site is also nearby.

Buffalo, with a population close to 300,000, is New York State's second-largest city. What makes it particularly appealing to the on-foot exerciser is its set of parks, based on the Buffalo Olmsted Park System, designed by Frederick Law Olmsted in the late 19th century. We chose to feature two parks, both reachable on-foot from downtown and of interest to both city visitors and residents.

Buffalo has more than its fair share of crime, with a statistic of 14.11 violent crimes per 1,000 inhabitants in 2006. However, we have seen no particular cause for concern about the routes we cover here, in daylight at least.

The focal point of Olmsted's original design, Delaware Park, has had a somewhat sad history. It was the venue for the 1901 Pan-America Exposition where President William McKinley was assassinated. The exposition's construction work badly damaged much of Olmsted's original design. Subsequently the park went into decline. Highway construction in the 1960s then added its toll to the park's environment.

Recently the Buffalo Olmsted Parks Conservancy has made major progress in reinstating what it can of Olmsted's plan. Delaware Park can today be considered the high point of Buffalo's park system, very popular with runners and walkers, plus golfers and other outdoor sportspeople.

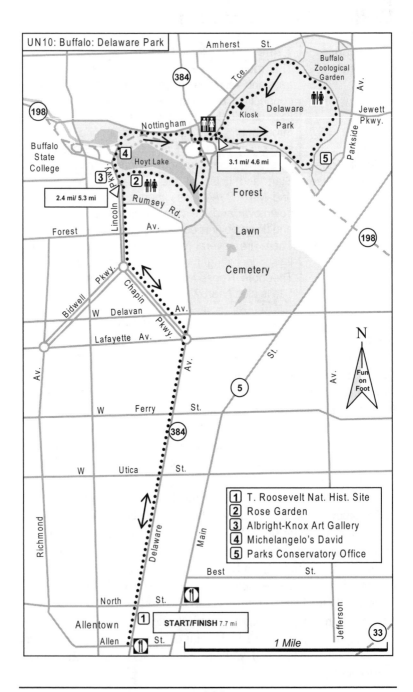

UN10: Buffalo: Delaware Park

Amherst St.

384

Buffalo Zoological Garden

Tce.

Av.

Nottingham

Kiosk

Delaware

Park

Jewett Pkwy.

198

Buffalo State College

4

Hoyt Lake

3.1 mi / 4.6 mi

Parkside

5

3

2

Forest

Lawn

Cemetery

198

2.4 mi / 5.3 mi

Rumsey Rd.

Av.

Lincoln Pkwy.

Forest

Av.

Bidwell

Pkwy.

Chapin

W Delavan

Av.

Lafayette Av.

Av.

Pkwy.

N

Fun
on
Foot

Av.

5

St.

Av.

W Ferry St.

384

W Utica St.

1 T. Roosevelt Nat. Hist. Site
2 Rose Garden
3 Albright-Knox Art Gallery
4 Michelangelo's David
5 Parks Conservatory Office

Richmond

Delaware

Main

Best St.

Jefferson

33

North St.

Allentown   1   **START/FINISH** 7.7 mi

Allen St.   1 Mile

Delaware Park is a little over three miles north of Buffalo's central business and government district, around Niagara Square and nearby Lafayette Square. The main life center of Buffalo is spread along a strip of roughly a mile from Lafayette Square north to Allentown. Hotels are also spread throughout that strip. We decided to feature Delaware Park plus the 2.4-mile connection to it from Allentown.

Delaware Park comprises two lobes, split apart by the highways Route 198 and Route 384. The east lobe is mostly a wide, open area containing an 18-hole golf course and sporting fields. It also has a loop road (with very limited traffic) and an accompanying jogging trail, making it very attractive to on-foot exercisers. The loop distance is approximately 1.5 miles.

The west lobe contains pretty Hoyt Lake, wooded terrain, and most of the remaining Olmsted features. There are various trails and a loop of the west lobe can be up to 1.4 miles.

We decided to put it all together, giving a 7.7-mile route comprising the sidewalk trip from Allentown plus loops of both park lobes. We have tried to do this in a way that makes it easy for you to pull the pieces apart and only do what best suits you.

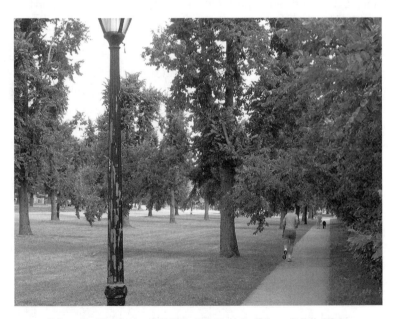

Lincoln Parkway: Wish All Roads Were Like This

To get between central downtown and Allentown (Allen Street), we recommend following Delaware Boulevard. Richmond Avenue, which runs parallel to Delaware Boulevard, was part of the original Olmsted design but is just not as nice as the latter today.

At Lafayette Avenue, bear left away from Delaware Boulevard onto Chapin Parkway, a wide thoroughfare which is part of Olmsted's design. At the next traffic circle, bear right along Lincoln Parkway. Parkways such as Chapin and Lincoln provide an outstanding on-foot environment, with excellent trails, virtually no vehicles, and a beautifully landscaped environment. Lincoln Parkway brings you to the southwest corner of Delaware Park, at Rumsey Road.

Pass the Elmwood Avenue Art Gallery on the left and the Lincoln statue on the right. Also on the right are also the Rose Garden and its Shakespeare-in-the-Park set, and the banquet venue called Marcy Casino. Continuing up Lincoln Parkway, cross the lake bridge and pass the copy of Michelangelo's Statue of David.

VARIATION

If you want to simply explore the west lobe of Delaware Park but not the east lobe, leave the street here and pick up the pedestrian trail around Hoyt Lake.

Take the pedestrian overpass over Route 198 and bear right on the pleasant trail following Nottingham Terrace, north of Route 198. Just before you get to the Delaware Avenue intersection (with the traffic lights), take the pedestrian sidewalk up the Route 198 exit ramp and go left around the sidewalk of the highway bridge. This brings you directly to the southwest corner of the east lobe of Delaware Park. There are restrooms here.

Pick up the east lobe loop trail here. You have a choice of using the road or a sinter-surface jogging track. While there are vehicles on parts of the road loop, they are limited to 15 mph and pedestrians freely use the road. On either trail, try to go counterclockwise, which most exercisers do. Expect to be in the company of many runners and walkers here, with cyclists in the minority.

The loop circumnavigates the golf course and sporting fields. On the east side, a little off the loop, is the Parks Conservancy office where you can find maps and information (weekdays only).

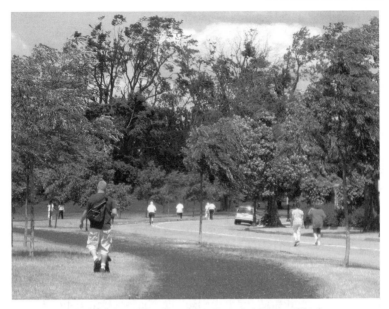

The Jogging Track or the Road—Your Choice

Pass the zoo and continue to the exit road onto Nottingham Terrace. There is a seasonal snack kiosk here. Continue back to where you started the loop, near the restrooms.

To return to the west lobe of the park, we can suggest a different route to how you came. Take the sidewalk of the bridge along Route 198 to the exit ramp. Then take the steps down to the west sidewalk of Delaware Avenue. Go under Route 198, cross two road ramps, and enter Delaware Park's west lobe. There are trails heading off both ways around Hoyt Lake. Choose either way. They both lead you back to the Rose Garden and Shakespeare set.

Retrace your steps to downtown Buffalo via Lincoln Parkway, Chapin Parkway, and Delaware Avenue. Alternatively, there is a subway service down Main Street a block east.

If you want a food or drink break, Allentown has much to offer. You can do no better than the famous Anchor Bar, credited with originating the concept of Buffalo Wings. When you reach North Street, go a block east to Main Street—the Anchor Bar is on the corner.

There are also several restaurants and pubs in Allen Street. Nola and I liked the Colter Bar and Grill at the intersection of Delaware Avenue and Allen Street—simple but friendly.

Buffalo: LaSalle Park

Distance	4.1 miles loop (Route UN11)
Comfort	This route involves a 1.7-mile loop on a good park trail. Add 1.2 miles each way from downtown to the park on a mixture of street sidewalks and pedestrian trails. Expect some other pedestrians around throughout. Inline skating is possible on parts of the route but not recommended overall.
Attractions	Escape to a pleasant lakeside park and enjoy the fresh air, away from city crowds and vehicles.
Convenience	Start and finish at Niagara Square, near the Buffalo Niagara Convention Center.
Destination	There are restaurants, bars, and stores near the finish.

This route is ideal for anyone working or staying in the Buffalo business and government district, or at the Buffalo Niagara Convention Center, and seeking a quick on-foot outing.

Start and finish at Niagara Square, the center of the business and government district. Go south down Niagara Street and bear right into Franklin Street. (If starting from the convention center, go straight down Franklin Street.) At the intersection with Erie Street and Swan Street, go right into Erie Street.

Erie Street takes you under Route 5 and under Interstate 190. Then take the paved trail to the right following the Interstate. The trail leads to LaSalle Park on the waterfront. Follow the trail along the water, past the outdoor entertainment venue and past the city water pumping station to Porter Avenue. This is a very pleasant, scenic path.

Return to where you entered the park by either going around the pumping station and following Dar Drive through the sporting fields or by retracing your steps on the trail along the water. Then return to downtown the same way you came.

On getting back to the downtown center, there are restaurants and pubs around the Main Street mall and Lafayette Square, three blocks east of Niagara Square.

VARIATION

You can follow Porter Avenue out of the park. It runs into North Street, which intersects Route UN10 (Buffalo: Delaware Park), allowing you to get to Allentown or Delaware Park. The problem with this route is that Porter Avenue tends to have very busy traffic coming from or going to the nearby Peace Bridge to Canada.

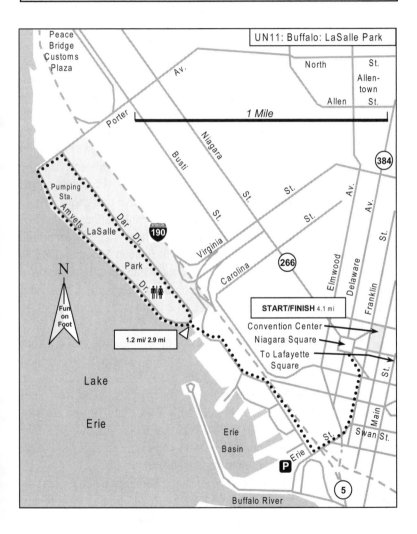

Other Routes

There are innumerable good running or walking routes in Upstate New York. Here are a few more suggestions of routes close to major centers that we have explored or have otherwise come to our attention.

In **Albany**, as well as our two featured routes, see the website www. hmrrc.com for a Spectator's Guide to the Mohawk Hudson River Marathon, which is effectively a walking tour of the riverside. There are other on-foot route ideas at www.albanyrunningexchange.org.

Beacon, near the east end of the Interstate 84 Hudson River bridge, has some trails that are easily accessed on-foot from the city center. The trails are quite well maintained and most have blazes, but the going is sometimes steep and the underfoot conditions stony and rough. Therefore, most people would hike rather than run these trails. Start at the intersection of Fishkill Avenue and Main Street. Go up Main Street, E Main Street, and then Pocket Street to the trailhead near the big city water tank. Follow the white-blazed trail to where it intersects the access road to Beacon Reservoir. You here have two choices (both roughly seven miles round-trip from the water tank trailhead). For the first choice, follow the access road up to the reservoir, go around the reservoir, and continue up the path to South Beacon Mountain and its fire tower. For the second choice, keep to the white blazed trail and do a loop of Fishkill Ridge. Both options provide excellent views in several different directions. After returning to the trailhead, continue back to the lively town.

The **Finger Lakes Trail** is a network of hiking trails in New York State. The main trail is 562 miles long and connects the Catskill Mountains in eastern New York with the Allegheny Mountains in southwestern New York at the Philadelphia border. The main trail passes through the southern region of New York State. If you are near the trail, you might want to use stretches of it for out-and-back trail running training. For more information and maps contact the Finger Lakes Trail Conference at www.fingerlakestrail.org.

Kingston was the first capital of New York State and is famous for having been razed by the British in the Revolution. It was rebuilt afterwards by its residents and is a fascinating historic destination today. Kingston has two main centers—the Stockade district and the Rondout district (by the waterfront), about 2.5 miles apart. Both districts are well worth visiting, making for a nice on-foot roundtrip, regardless of where you start. The main connecting road between the two districts, Broadway, is not exciting but has good sidewalks and traverses a quite respectable area. There are great food and beverage places in both end districts. Do not miss the Hoffman House Tavern in the Stockade district—the building, ambiance, and food quality are outstanding. When asked about running routes, the local visitor information centers pointed us to the D&H Canal Heritage Corridor, but they were vague on details. Under this project, a substantial trail system, combining rail-trail segments and canal towpaths, is planned and some parts are in place. However, the trail segment we eventually found connecting to central Kingston was in very poor shape, and we cannot recommend it today. To explore the D&H Canal Heritage Corridor, you would need to drive out of Kingston, and you should check on the latest trail status before doing that.

In **Niagara Falls** you will find the nation's most spectacular on-foot route—the Goat Island loop. From 1st Street and Rainbow Boulevard, head south across the bridge to Goat Island. Go left, around the very pleasant island. The eastern part of the island has few tourists and considerable birdlife. Follow the paved trail, with excellent views of the flowing waters all around the island. Optionally divert on the short path to the Three Sisters Islands. On getting near the falls, take the lower walkway to Terrapin Point and the Horseshoe Falls. The Horseshoe Falls are breathtaking close up, but you may encounter crowds of tourists around here. Go up the trail past the Top of the Falls Restaurant. You can then divert to Luna Island between the little Bridal Veil Falls and the American Falls. Take the bridge to Green Island and on to the mainland. Go left to the end of the American Falls, with more excellent views along here. Finish back in the city center.

Also in Niagara Falls, the trail upstream from the falls is excellent. Do an out and back loop from the city center on this paved trail along the fast flowing river.

If you are visiting **Poughkeepsie** and staying in a hotel on Route 9 near the IBM campus, there are some good running places nearby but you generally need to drive to them. Roughly a mile north of IBM is the **Samuel Morse Historic Site**, a National Historic Landmark. It has about three miles of carriage roads traversing a beautifully landscaped park. Better still, if you are prepared to drive four miles, you can get to 301-acre **Bowdoin Park**. It has some great trails, some with scenic Hudson River views. The park includes a marked 5K cross-country course. Drive south on Route 9 to Sheafe Road, off to the right about 1.5 miles from IBM. The park is 2.5 miles down Sheafe Road.

Here are more suggestions around Poughkeepsie: the Staatsburgh State Historic Site with connections to Norrie State Park; Vassar College Farm; Minnewaska State Park Preserve, New Paltz; Wallkill River Rail Trail, New Paltz; Harlem Valley Rail Trail, Amenia; and Tymor Forest Park near Union Vale.

Rhinebeck is a lively, historic town just off the Hudson's east bank. It is popular with New Yorkers as a country retreat. Nola and I spent a memorable night and day there, staying in the 1766-vintage Beekman Arms which claims to be "America's oldest inn." We hunted hard for good local runs, without much success, except for short jogs around the town streets. The visitor center provided a brochure on "Bike and Walk Tour." However, the routes suggested involved much use of the edges of country roads that carry substantial traffic. We therefore hesitate to recommend these.

Near **Rochester**, we featured the most popular section of the Genesee Riverway trail, south of the city, in Route UN9 (Rochester: Genesee Riverway). The Genesee Riverway also extends north of the city, connecting Rochester and Lake Ontario. At the time of writing, the trail is completed from Lower Falls Park about two miles north of the city, through Olmsted-designed Maplewood Park, and Turning Point Park to the lakeshore. Parts of the route are multiuse trails and parts follow streets. Further trail extensions and improvements are planned. For latest status refer to the website of the City of Rochester Parks and Recreation Department.

Also Rochester has a paved trail, the **Canalway Trail**, following the Erie Canal for several miles. You can access this trail in the west and east directions at Genesee Valley Park, the southern end of Route UN9 (Rochester: Genesee Riverway). In the west direction, the trail extends to Tonawanda, near Buffalo but it is mostly unpaved and of varying quality. For more information consult the website www.nyscanals. gov.

Saratoga Spa State Park is near **Saratoga Springs**, just south of downtown between Routes 9 and 50. It has several miles of walking, running, and hiking trails, plus some paved roads suitable for running.

There is a cross-country course—see www.saratogastryders.org for a map. There is more information on the park at www.saratogastatepark. org. There is also running (including a marked 5K course) at Camp Saratoga, part of the Wilton Wildlife Preserve and Park; see www. saratogastryders.org.

Schenectady is a city on the Mohawk River, along the route of the Mohawk-Hudson Bike-Hike Trail. From downtown Schenectady, you can do an interesting three-mile loop around a segment of the river, making use of different segments of that trail. From downtown Schenectady, go north up N Jay Street, past South Avenue, to the start of the rail-trail. Follow the trail to the access point at Seneca Street. Leave the trail here and head northwest to the river, following the road. Cross the river on the bridge sidewalk. Across the river, pick up another trail segment heading back upstream. It brings you to Collins Park in the town of Scotia, across the river from Schenectady. There are seasonal restrooms in the park. Then follow the sidewalk of the Route 5 Western Gateway Bridge back to downtown Schenectady.

For **Syracuse** we featured the city's on-foot gem, Onondaga Lake Park, in route UN8 (Syracuse: Onondaga Lake Park). Another interesting route, especially for someone staying downtown, is the **Creekwalk**. This trail extends from the northwest corner of downtown through the Franklin Park area to Inner Harbor and further west. There is much development going on around this part of Syracuse, rejuvenating the area. Hopefully this will ultimately lead to the linking of the Creekwalk to the Carousel Center and on to Onondaga Lake Park.

Other trails around Syracuse include Pratt's Falls Park and Highland Forest County Park, southeast of the city, a short drive away. There is also good running on the roads and streets southeast of the Syracuse University campus, including Meadowbrook Drive, and in Green Lakes State Park and Beaver Lake County Park.

Running Clubs

Albany: Albany Running Exchange (www.albanyrunningexchange. org)

Formed in the fall of 2002, the Albany Running Exchange is a unique organization that offers numerous daily group runs, limitless social events including weekend retreats and Caribbean cruises, and an interactive members page that promotes camaraderie and communication. Members range in age from 7 to 73 with a full spectrum of abilities. Email: Refer to website

Albany: Hudson-Mohawk Road Runners Club (www.hmrrc.com)

The Hudson-Mohawk Road Runners Club has over 2,000 members. Members come in all shapes and sizes and from all walks of life, as well as different running styles and speeds. All are united in a love of running and a desire to promote and participate in quality races and running-related activities. The club organizes nearly 30 running events a year. Club races are held at many different locations throughout the Capital District. Club events offer something for everyone, novice and veteran alike. Email: mjkhome@verizon.net

Amsterdam: Fulmont Road Runners (www.fmrrc.org)

This club welcomes all levels of runners. Members come from a wide area of Montgomery and Fulmont Counties. Email: Refer to website

Binghamton: Triple Cities Runners Club (www.triplecitiesrunnersclub.org)

This club, formed about 20 years ago, has approximately 240 members. It welcomes all levels of runners. It sponsors many races throughout the year and provides finish-line services for 20-25 races per year. Email: Refer to website

Buffalo: Checkers Athletic Club (www.checkersac.org)

With a firm commitment to "fitness, health, and well-being for life," this club services a membership of approximately 500 runners from Western New York and Southern Ontario. Checkers' members go on the road to participate in marathons, cross-country meets, and indoor track events. The club sponsors several local races, including the Checkers Mile in May in Lockport NY, the Checkers Tavern Pie Race, the Ring-Road

Relay, and a High School Cross Country Invitational in November for the top scholastic athletes in Western New York. The club also hosts monthly and annual social events including happy hours, fun runs, a summer picnic, and a holiday party.
Email: webmaster@checkersac.org

Buffalo: Nickel City Road Runners (www.nickelcityroadrunners. com)
The club has monthly happy hours, a holiday party, summer picnics, weekly runs, and other events throughout the year. Members run and walk from the Ken-Ton YMCA on Belmont Avenue near Sheridan Drive, Town of Tonawanda, every Tuesday evening. After running and walking, members meet for dinner and drinks. There are monthly meetings on the first Tuesday of the month.
Email: Refer to website

Glens Falls: Adirondack Runners Club (www.adirondackrunners. com)
This club has 400-to-500 members and welcomes all levels of runners. It covers the greater Glens Falls area, including Queensbury and Lake George. The club meets for running on Sunday mornings and Wednesday evenings and has a monthly meeting. It sponsors seven premier races during the year. Its Scholarship Fund makes awards at the end of each school year in a continuing effort to promote youth development.
Email: Refer to website

Ithaca: The Finger Lakes Runners Club (www.fingerlakesrunners. org)
The Finger Lakes Runners Club provides educational, informational, and community services, in order to promote fitness and health through running. The club holds a variety of competitive and noncompetitive events, such as track meets, road races, and cross-country or trail runs. Consult the club's website for running route ideas in the vicinity of Ithaca and Trumansburg.
Email: board@fingerlakesrunners.org

Onteora: Onteora Runners Club (www.onteorarunners.org)
The club is located in the Mid-Hudson Valley of New York State, in the shadow of the Catskill Mountains, and currently has around 400 members. The mission is to promote running and fitness for runners of all

ages. The club offers individual and family memberships. It holds numerous fun runs including winter breakfast runs and weekday summer trail runs. The club sponsors a group of races at varied distances, from a mile race on the track, to a 10.5-mile race on single-track trails, and a yearly competitive Grand Prix series followed by an awards banquet. Email: orc.prez@yahoo.com

Orange County: Orange Runners Club (www.orangerunnersclub. org)
This club supports and encourages runners of all ages and levels of experience. You may run to lose weight; achieve or maintain fitness; complete or win road races; enjoy the outdoors in a free and unencumbered way; or experience the inner strength, growth, and higher level of self-esteem that comes from meeting and exceeding your goals. Whatever your reasons, this club is ready to share years of combined experiences (and war stories), insight and endless amounts of enthusiasm. The club is committed to supporting healthy, injury-free running, and of course, fun.
Email: Refer to website

Rochester: Genesee Valley Harriers Running Club (www.gvh.net)
The main goal of this club is to field full and competitive teams (male, female and masters) for regional and national competitions in cross country, road racing, and track events. Simultaneously, the Genesee Valley Harriers Running Club (GVH) wants to help promote individual achievement and success on a year-round basis. Additionally, GVH sponsors and supports running related activities throughout the community. GVH desires to have all of its members strive for excellence and to be involved in all club activities. These include team races, team workouts, Sunday long runs, club meeting and social gatherings.
Email: coachmr@rochester.rr.com or pglavin@rochester.rr.com

Rochester: Greater Rochester Track Club (www.grtconline.org)
The Greater Rochester Track Club (GRTC) is a not-for-profit, volunteer organization that was founded in 1955. It is one of the oldest and largest organized running clubs in the North East. GRTC has approximately 500 members, consisting of runners, walkers, athletes, and fitness enthusiasts, encompassing an eight county region. The club's goals are to help you be more fit, help you learn more about yourself, and provide information to help prevent common running injuries. So, whether you

are a jogger or a runner, ready to race or someone keeping in shape, GRTC membership is for you.
Email: Refer to website

Rome: The Roman Runners (www.romanrunners.com)
This is a club of 150 members ranging in age from 10 to 94. The club sponsors about 10 races per year, has weekly training runs, an annual awards banquet, bus trips to races, and many social gatherings. At New Years, some club members traditionally do a three-race sequence in Saratoga Springs, New York City, and Rome, involving 13.3 miles on foot and 12 hours on a bus, all in 17 hours.
Email: Refer to website

Saratoga Springs: Saratoga Stryders (www.saratogastryders.org)
Established in 1984, the goal of this club is to promote fitness through running and related sports, to educate the community about the benefits of these activities, and to provide a bond for both serious and recreational runners. Membership includes all ages and abilities, and the program is broad enough to accommodate the interests of everyone—from beginning walkers and runners to veteran marathoners. The club has Saturday morning runs year-round in Saratoga Spa State Park. Runners divide into groups according to pace/distance and most run about an hour on trails and paved roads within the park. There are also Wednesday evening workouts and the club hosts races and social events.
Email: info@saratogastryders.org

Syracuse: Syracuse Chargers Track Club (www.syracusechargers. org)
This club is forty years old in 2009. The all-volunteer organization encourages regular participation in track and field (indoor and outdoor), road running, cross-country running, trail running, and race walking by people of all ages and levels of interest and ability. The club conducts more than fifty organized events annually, with three-quarters of them free for members and non-members alike. In addition, the club maintains a website; publishes a monthly newsletter; supports competitive teams and post-collegiate athletic development; conducts an annual college scholarship program; and conducts year-round programs for non-competitive runners and walkers as well as developmentally disabled individuals.
Email: daveoja@festivalofraces.com

Ticonderoga: La Chute Road Runners (www.lachute.us)
This club in northeastern New York State encourages the youth of the community to get involved in a beneficial activity, provides competitive opportunities for its membership, and provides membership with educational and social opportunities. The club sponsors the Montcalm Mile, the Resolution Run, and the Heritage Day 10K. It also supports a Point Championship Series, holds an annual awards banquet, provides a newsletter, and provides organized training opportunities.
Email: Refer to website

Utica: Utica Roadrunners (www.uticaroadrunners.org)
The club motto is: "A place for every pace." Whether you are running one mile per week or 100, racing at five minutes per mile pace or 15, there is a place for you in the Utica Roadrunners. There are monthly meetings, fun runs, a Boilermaker Training Program, summer and fall development runs, an annual holiday party, an annual awards banquet, and a Grand Prix race series. The club also organizes several local races.
Email: Refer to website

11

Some New Jersey Gems

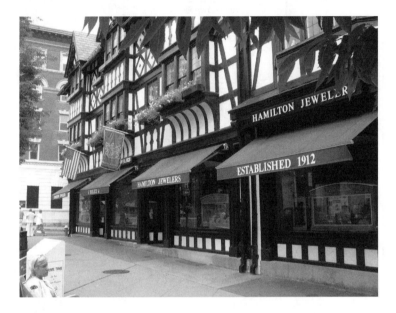

B efore New Jersey locals start feeling offended, let me hasten
to point out that New Jersey is in no way part of New York.
However, residents of and visitors to the greater New York City
region and New Jersey intermingle so much we cannot ignore New
Jersey on-foot routes in this book.[1]

In Chapter 7 we covered the strip of New Jersey on the Hudson
bank, immediately across from Manhattan. For routes in Hoboken,
Jersey City, Liberty State Park, and Palisades Park, see that chapter. In
this chapter, we feature six outstanding on-foot routes near New Jersey
centers a little further away from the Big Apple.

---

1   Chapter head photo: Charming downtown Princeton, NJ.

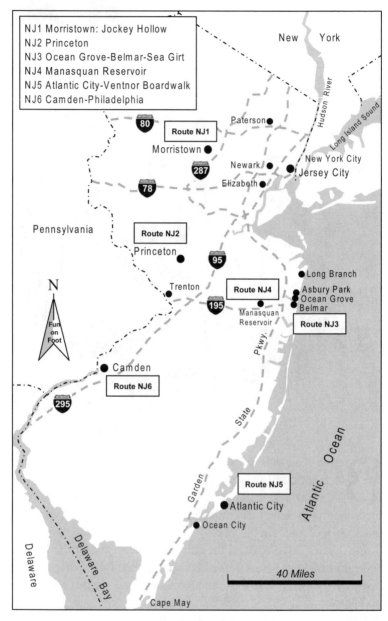

NJ1 Morristown: Jockey Hollow
NJ2 Princeton
NJ3 Ocean Grove-Belmar-Sea Girt
NJ4 Manasquan Reservoir
NJ5 Atlantic City-Ventnor Boardwalk
NJ6 Camden-Philadelphia

New Jersey Routes

Route	Distance
NJ1 Morristown: Jockey Hollow	Various
NJ2 Princeton	5.4 miles loop
NJ3 Ocean Grove-Belmar-Sea Girt	6.2 miles one way
NJ4 Manasquan Reservoir	5.1 miles loop
NJ5 Atlantic City-Ventnor Boardwalk	3.6 miles one way
NJ6 Camden-Philadelphia	4.3 miles one way

In the Other Routes section that follows the featured route descriptions, we summarize some additional route ideas.

Morristown: Jockey Hollow

Distance	Various (Route NJ1)
Comfort	Unpaved pedestrian trails of varying quality, ranging from well-maintained earth trails to trails that are quite rugged and rocky. Some people run these trails but that can be hazardous. There are also paved roads that are quite pedestrian-friendly. Expect to meet other people on the trails, but no crowds. Inline skating is neither practical nor permitted.
Attractions	Historic sites and recreations.
Convenience	Start and finish at either the Visitor Center or Trail Center of the Jockey Hollow Area. There is parking at both locations.
Destination	If you have not done so before, see the displays at the Visitor Center explaining the local history.

What makes Morristown special is the Morristown National Historic Park. This park preserves the history of the area where Washington and his Continental Army camped for two winters in the late 1770s. The soldiers lived under extreme conditions, particularly in the winter of 1779-1780. The park comprises three sites—the Ford Mansion, Fort Nonsense, and Jockey Hollow. The first two of these sites are quite small and in easy walking distance of downtown Morristown. Jockey Hollow is a few miles further southwest of downtown. While all these places are well worth seeing, Jockey Hollow is the one place that offers an excellent opportunity for good-distance on-foot exercise, combined with a peaceful woodland environment and historic sites in abundance to help keep the mind active.

There is a substantial trail network in the park, with the major trails being color-blazed. The main loop trails are:

- White Trail (Grand Loop Trail): Approximately 5.5 miles;
- Blue Trail (New York Brigade Trail, Mount Kemble Loop Trail, and Old Camp Road Trail): Approximately three miles;

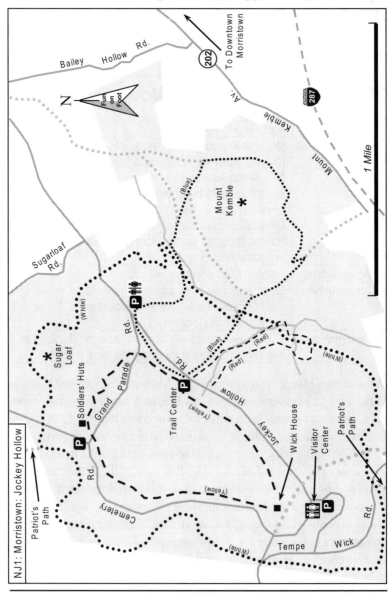

- Yellow Trail (Soldier Hut Trail and Grand Parade Trail): Approximately two miles;
- Red Trail (Primrose Brook Trail): Approximately one mile.

These trails vary from earth, with gravel in parts, to rocky requiring care. After substantial rains, parts of the trails may become waterlogged. Bikes, inline skating, and off-leash pets are prohibited. Maps are posted at major trail intersections so it is difficult to get lost. If doing the White trail, be careful when crossing Tempe Wick Road since vehicles travel quite fast on that road.

Another option is to walk or run around the paved "tour road" and many people do just that. This involves the loop of Cemetery Road, Grand Parade Road, and Jockey Hollow Road. Vehicle traffic on this loop is very light and travels slowly.

You need to drive to Jockey Hollow. Pick up a trail map at the Visitor Center and park either there or at the Trail Center. The latter location is not really a center; just a car park, but it is handy to most of the trails. There is also a third parking lot near the Soldiers' Huts.

The Patriots' Path, a hiking trail network spanning much of southern Morris County, also passes through this area. For more detail consult the website www.morrisparks.org.

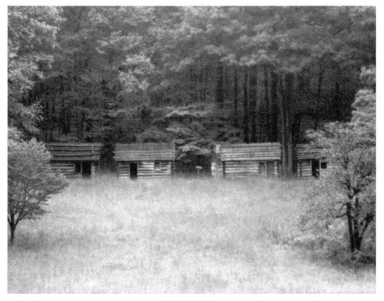

The Soldiers' Huts

Princeton

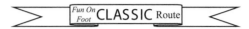

Distance	6.4 miles loop (Route NJ2)
Comfort	Dedicated pedestrian trails, some paved and some earth, with a few sections along street sidewalks. There are few vehicle-traffic interruptions. Not recommended overall for inline skating.
Attractions	Traverse the Princeton University campus and do a very pleasant loop along scenic Carnegie Lake and the historic Delaware and Raritan Canal.
Convenience	Start and finish in the heart of Princeton at the main entrance to campus, adjacent to the town center.
Destination	There are several restaurants, bars and shops in the town center.

Princeton is a very pleasant campus community in a beautiful environment. The campus is sandwiched between the quaint town center and the watercourses of Carnegie Lake and the Delaware and Raritan Canal. The latter is now managed as the Delaware and Raritan Canal State Park. The lake and canal serve as a playground for rowing, kayaking, cycling, running, and walking.

This is a low-crime town (1.55 violent crimes per 1,000 inhabitants in 2006).

We decided to feature one loop route that includes the campus, the lake, and the canal. This is an outstanding route in its own right, but also consider it an introduction to the neighborhood, helping you to craft your own routes afterwards.

The natural center of Princeton is the intersection of Nashua Street and Witherspoon Street, adjacent to the Princeton Borough center at Palmer Square and across from the Front Campus entrance to Princeton University. We nominally start our featured route there.

Enter the campus and work your way south. For example, from the Front Campus entrance, bear right around Nassau Hall, skirt Cannon Green, and pick up Elm Drive, which weaves southward. Admire the beautiful Princeton architecture. When you get down to the softball field, follow the paved pedestrian trail peeling off to the left before the tennis center.

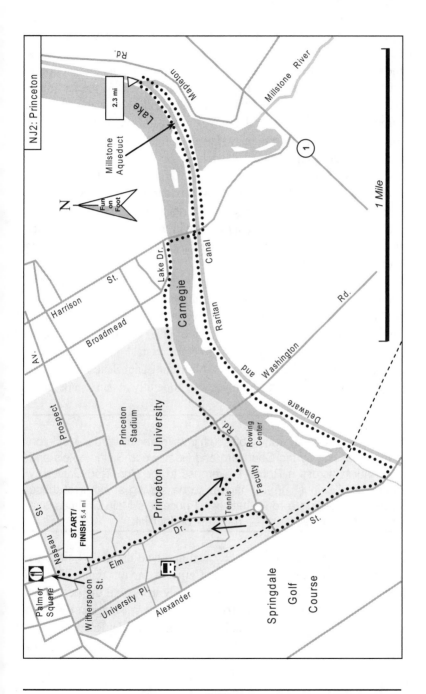

When the path emerges at Faculty Road, go left along the paved trail following that road to the intersection with Washington Road. Cross Washington Road and continue on the trail about 150 yards to the car parking access point across the road. Go into that little parking area, which is popular with kayakers and canoeists. At the far end of the parking area, there is a small trailhead. Follow a lovely earth trail through the trees, to where it emerges at Broadmead and Lake Drive. Follow quiet Lake Drive to busy Harrison Street, and go right, crossing Lake Carnegie on the bridge sidewalk.

You then come to the Delaware and Raritan Canal. The canal was built as a route for freighting goods between Philadelphia and New York, connecting the Delaware and Raritan Rivers. Today there are paths on both sides of the canal here, with the path on the north side being wide and well maintained, and the path on the south side being narrower and less used.

We suggest doing a loop eastward to the Millstone Aqueduct and footbridge. Cross the canal on the Harrison Street bridge and follow the canal to the left. You are now in a very peaceful, almost wilderness environment, although there are plenty of other outdoor lovers not far away. Cross the aqueduct when you come to it. You then come to a formal entrance to the Delaware and Raritan Canal State Park, with a map sign and a box from which you can hopefully obtain a paper map.

VARIATION

There is a trail heading off south from this point, across Mapleton Road, passing by the Courtyard and Homewood Suites hotels and continuing across a Route 1 overpass to the Princeton University Forrestal Campus. If you happen to be staying at either of these hotels or seeking a route between Princeton's Main Campus and Forrestal Campus, here you have the on-foot link.

Cross the footbridge over the canal and take the main trail to the left back along the canal, with Lake Carnegie on your right. This is a beautiful trail, with water both sides, shady trees, and the occasional canoeist or kayaker. Cross Harrison Street and Washington Road, go under the rail track overpass, and emerge on Alexander Road.

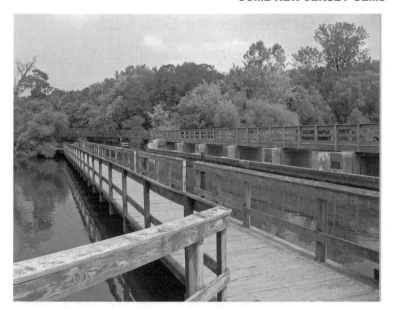

Pedestrian Bridges over the Millstone Aqueduct

VARIATION

If you want to extend your outing with an out-and-back segment, continue further on the canal trail and return back here. Alternatively, if you want to get to the Hyatt Regency Hotel, go south down Alexander Road and across Route 1.

To return to the Princeton campus or downtown, follow the trail up Alexander Road (which becomes Alexander Street) to the Faculty Road intersection. From here you can follow Faculty Road to the Elm Drive rotary and Elm Drive back to our route's start point. You could equally well take the trail up Alexander Street to University Place and then follow University Place up to Nassau Street.

If you need a food or beverage break, there are several fine choices around Palmer Square.

Ocean Grove-Belmar-Sea Girt

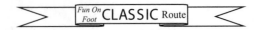

Distance	6.2 miles one way (Route NJ3)
Comfort	This route is almost entirely on boardwalks and paved trails along the ocean shore. There are no vehicle traffic interruptions. Expect plenty of other on-foot exercisers around. Inline skating is prohibited on much of the route, except early morning (rules vary along the route).
Attractions	Beautiful ocean and beach views the entire route. Plenty of fresh air.
Convenience	Start at Main Avenue and the Boardwalk in Ocean Grove and finish at Trenton Boulevard and the Boardwalk in Sea Girt. It is less than a half-mile from either of these points to a connecting bus route along Route 71. There are many options to park and do out-and-back segments or to reverse the basic route.
Destination	There are wind-down food and beverage establishments at both ends of this route.

This route is one of the most perfect ocean-side trails you will find anywhere. It involves a six-mile uninterrupted run along a mix of boardwalks and paved trails, in an environment where crowds are unlikely to be a problem. You can do this route equally well either direction, as an out-and-back route or a one-way journey with a bus return.[2]

There is a bus route that services points along this route—it roughly follows Route 71, less than a half-mile inland. There is also a rail line following this route, generally tracking Route 71 and ultimately connecting to New York City. This is the NJ Transit North Jersey Coast Line. Therefore, for someone living in or visiting New York City, this route is comparatively easy to work into your plans.

We decided to fix the northern end of our route at Main Avenue, Ocean Grove. The boardwalk continues a little further north of here to Asbury Park, a mile away. However, Asbury Park has such a bad

---

2   Thanks to Greg Mulligan and Joe Hornyak for recommending this route to us.

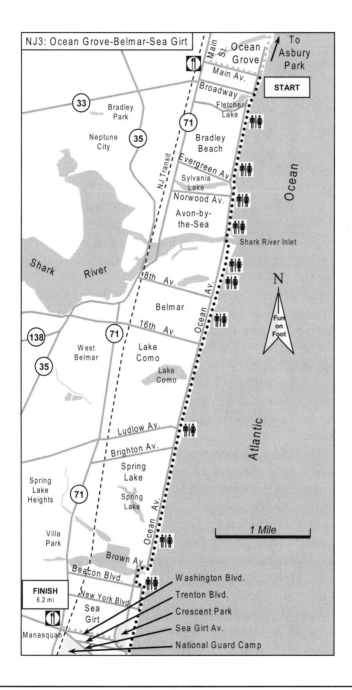

NJ3: Ocean Grove-Belmar-Sea Girt

Main St.

Ocean Grove

To Asbury Park

Main Av.

Broadway

START

33

Bradley Park

Fletcher Lake

71

Neptune City

35

Bradley Beach

NJ Transit

Evergreen Av.

Sylvania Lake

Norwood Av.

Avon-by-the-Sea

Ocean

Shark River Inlet

Shark River

18th Av.

Ocean Av.

N

Belmar

138

West Belmar

16th Av.

Fun on Foot

71

Lake Como

35

Lake Como

Ludlow Av.

Atlantic

Brighton Av.

Spring Lake Heights

Spring Lake

71

Spring Lake

Ocean Av.

1 Mile

Villa Park

Brown Av.

Beacon Blvd.

FINISH
6.2 mi

New York Blvd.

Washington Blvd.

Sea Girt

Trenton Blvd.

Crescent Park

Manasquan

Sea Girt Av.

National Guard Camp

reputation (including a quite alarming statistic of 23.2 violent crimes per 1,000 inhabitants in 2006) we did not want to encourage our readers to go there. Asbury Park is unquestionably improving itself, with major reconstruction projects underway. However, it is a different world to Ocean Grove, a beautiful little place with a lovely beach and a charming main street packed with antique stores and other small businesses.

Ocean Grove is a dry town. However, if you seek an alcoholic beverage on finishing an on-foot route here, simply go up Main Avenue to Main Street (Route 71) and cross that street to Clancy's Tavern in Neptune City. It is an Irish pub with a great menu and a big local following.

We start our route at the Boardwalk in Ocean Grove, at Main Avenue. Head south down the Boardwalk. On this part of the route you are always on either a boardwalk or paved path, with vehicle traffic sufficiently far away. In summer months, bicycles and inline skates are prohibited after 10:00 am.

At Fletcher Lake you leave Ocean Grove and enter Bradley Beach. At Evergreen Avenue, which follows the edge of Sylvania Lake, you enter Avon-by-the-Sea. Between this point and Norwood Avenue there is a break in the boardwalk that forces you onto the street sidewalk but the going is still good.

As you get near the Shark River drawbridge, you are forced to move again to the street sidewalk and cross the drawbridge. This bridge crosses a busy waterway and is raised quite frequently so you may have to wait here.

You are now in Belmar, where the boardwalk restarts. Bicycles and inline skating are prohibited here year-round after 9:00 am. At 8th Avenue there is a grocery store and a couple of food joints. Where Lake Como meets the ocean, there is a break in the boardwalk for a short distance and you must use the sidewalk again.

After the Ludlow Avenue beach pavilion, the boardwalk separates from the road. Dogs and inline skating are prohibited on this section of the boardwalk at all times. The environment becomes quiet residential.

At Brown Avenue the boardwalk is interrupted and the road turns inland. Follow it around and go over a small bridge. You enter the borough of Sea Girt here. Go on to Beacon Boulevard and go left, to

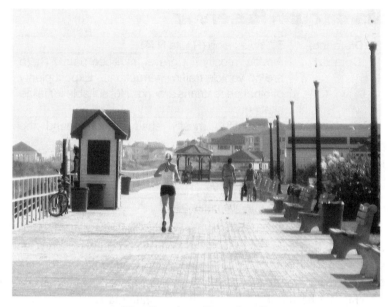

The Spacious Boardwalk

where the boardwalk starts again. Pass the Sea Girt lighthouse here and appreciate the beautiful homes that are characteristic of Sea Girt.

At New York Boulevard the road shifts away from the sea behind the houses but the boardwalk continues along the beach. Follow the boardwalk to its end at Trenton Boulevard—there is no shore access further south of here because of a US Military Reservation. Take Trenton Boulevard and Sea Girt Avenue or Washington Boulevard to Route 71 where they meet. At Route 71 there are some pubs, restaurants, and other services. There is also a bus stop here for NJ Transit services back to Ocean Grove and Asbury Park. There is rail service at Manasquan, a little south of here.

Manasquan Reservoir

Distance	5.1 miles loop (Route NJ4)
Comfort	A wide, mostly flat gravel, multiuse path. There are no vehicle traffic interruptions. Expect plenty of other pedestrians around. Not suitable for inline skating.
Attractions	A beautiful, mostly shady path around the reservoir.
Convenience	Start and finish at the Manasquan Reservoir visitor center, off Route 9 near Exit 28B of Interstate 195. There is parking here.
Destination	No specific destination.

This is a well-maintained and popular exercise trail. To get to the visitor center, take Interstate 195 Exit 28B to Route 9 north. Go right on Georgia Tavern Road and then right on Windeler Road to the visitor center entrance road. After parking, follow the signs to the Perimeter Trail.

This is a beautiful 5.1-mile loop, with mile markers. The path is wide and mostly under shady trees. The section along Georgia Tavern Road is the least pleasant owing to the nearby vehicle traffic. The trail is mostly flat, with a small hill around the 4.5-mile mark. There are

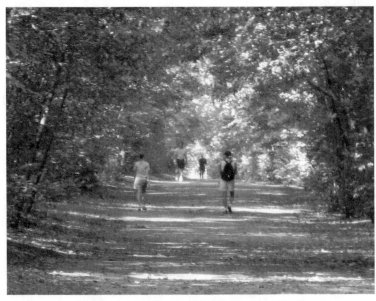

Manasquan Reservoir Perimeter Trail

restrooms at the visitor center, the environmental center, and Chestnut Point. Expect the company of other walkers, runners, and some bikes.

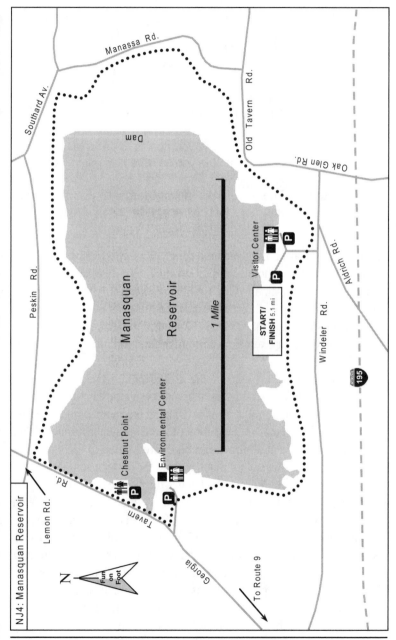

Atlantic City-Ventnor Boardwalk

Distance	3.6 miles one way (Route NJ5)
Comfort	This is an excellent quality route, on a boardwalk the entire way. Expect plenty of other pedestrians around. Mornings are best, to avoid the risk of crowds. Not recommended for inline skating.
Attractions	A beautiful ocean-side environment, in a very popular part of New Jersey.
Convenience	Start in the center of Atlantic City's tourist and gaming heart, at Park Place and the Boardwalk. We recommend you do this route as an out-and-back trip, unless you have vehicle return transport arranged.
Destination	There is no compelling destination at the south end but plenty of enjoyable destinations if you return to Atlantic City.

Atlantic City is an exciting vacation destination. It offers beautiful long sandy beaches, great hotels, and, of course, a good collection of gambling casinos. But Atlantic City is not a Las Vegas. Atlantic City truly does have family appeal, with activities for all ages from kids through young adults to baby boomers and beyond. Furthermore, it does have an excellent outdoor exercise environment, an attribute where Las Vegas fails miserably.

Outdoor activity centers on the Boardwalk. The Atlantic City Boardwalk is four miles long, and it connects seamlessly to the Ventnor Boardwalk, an additional 1.5 miles. There are quarter-mile markers the entire length, thanks to the efforts of the Boardwalk Runners Club. Dogs are prohibited at all times and bikes are limited to early morning hours. Therefore, this is very much a place for on-foot activity.

The nature of the Boardwalk changes during the day. In the mornings you will find many serious exercisers here, including good numbers of walkers, runners, and cyclists. Later in the day the scene changes. The Boardwalk is taken over by strolling, mostly-unfit tourists. What is really weird is the concept of chair-rides—this is a system where unfit people pay cash to fit people to push them in a wheeled chair along the Boardwalk. Handicapped persons aside, this is a really strange concept. The person pushing the chair is a double winner (gaining both fitness and money) while those in the chairs are double losers.

We feature the best part of the Boardwalk—the part from central Atlantic City heading south through Ventnor to the Margate City line.

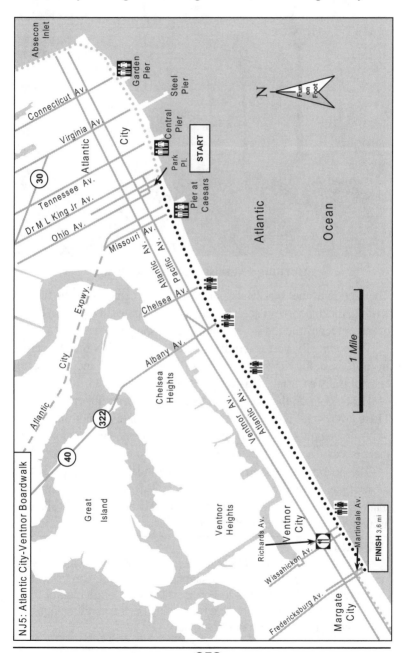

NJ5: Atlantic City-Ventnor Boardwalk

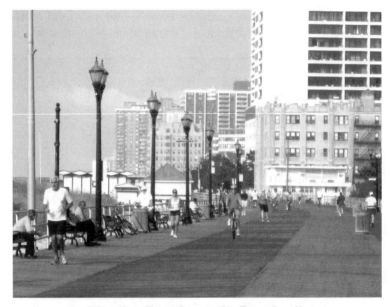

Morning Exercise on the Boardwalk

The section of the Boardwalk north of the city center is, at the time of writing, much poorer in quality. However, Atlantic City is in the throes of major reconstruction so that may change some time soon.

We nominally start where Park Place meets the Boardwalk, across from the tasteful New Jersey Korean War Memorial and the not-so-tasteful Bally's Casino. This is close to mile marker 2.25.

Head south on the Boardwalk, enjoying its beautiful environment. There are several restrooms along the way. There are not many food or beverage outlets until you get to Richards Avenue in Ventnor, where there is a café a short block in from the shore.

The boardwalk ends in Ventnor at Martindale Avenue, just before the Margate line at Fredericksburg Avenue. This is shortly after mileage marker 5.75. For a 7.2-mile return trip entirely on the Boardwalk, turn around here and go back to the start.

VARIATION

To continue on into Margate City, leave the Boardwalk at Martindale Avenue and go inland to Atlantic Avenue. You can follow the sidewalk of Atlantic Avenue to Longport Point (mileage marker 9.0). The sidewalk is quite reasonable for running but the surroundings are much less attractive than the Boardwalk.

Camden-Philadelphia

Distance	4.3 miles one way (Route NJ6)
Comfort	This route starts with good pedestrian paths on the Camden side followed by the Benjamin Franklin Bridge walkway. Pedestrians might be sparse on this part of the route at off-peak times but you could encounter crowds if you hit a special event. In Philadelphia, the route uses street sidewalks. Expect many other pedestrians around for that part. Inline skating is possible but challenging owing to the grades on the bridge and the pedestrian traffic in Philadelphia.
Attractions	Pass by Philadelphia's most historic sites, including Independence Hall, the Liberty Bell pavilion, Christ Church Burial Ground, and the Philadelphia Mint. See impressive views of the Delaware River and surrounds while crossing the Benjamin Franklin suspension bridge. Have a pleasant and scenic ferry ride back across the Delaware River. Finish at the New Jersey State Aquarium.
Convenience	Start at the New Jersey State Aquarium near Federal Street and Delaware Avenue, close to downtown Camden. Finish at Penn's Landing, directly across the river. You can catch a ferry from that finish point back to the start point.
Destination	There are many interesting sights, activities, restaurants, and bars around Penn's Landing. If you take the ferry back, you can visit the New Jersey State Aquarium and Walt Whitman House.

The city of Camden, in the southwest corner of New Jersey, has one attribute that makes it particularly exciting—it is a short hop across the Delaware River from Philadelphia, one of the nation's most vibrant and history-soaked cities. If you live in or visit Camden, here is an on-foot route you must not miss.

This route takes you along the river on the Camden side on a quality pedestrian trail and then across the river on the walkway/bikeway of the Benjamin Franklin Bridge. Once in Philadelphia you pass some of the most historic sites in the nation in Independence National Historic

Park, then the colorful and historic Society Hill area, and you finish at exciting Penn's Landing. From there you can catch a ferry back to your start point, but you might well choose to have a food or beverage stop in Philadelphia first.

This route may take longer than you would think, because of the ferry wait (not to mention the food and beverage stop). It is not a serious

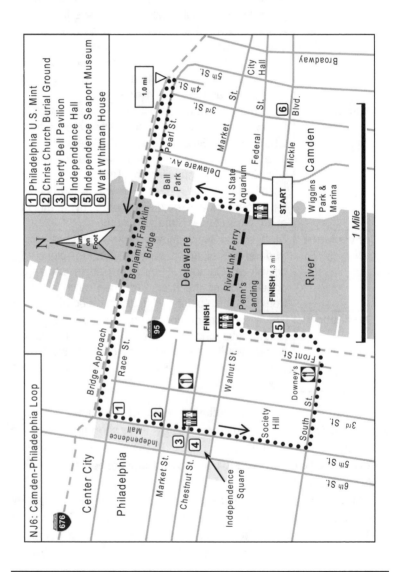

training route for marathoners, but it sure makes for a very pleasant afternoon out.

Starting from the aquarium, find the riverfront trail heading northward towards the Benjamin Franklin Bridge. Proceed up to and past Campbell's Field, the junior league ballpark. Go right along Pearl Street to North 4th Street. Here you find stairs that take you up to the bridge's southern walkway.

The grade up the bridge is significant but the easy downhill that follows compensates for that. All in all, crossing the bridge on foot is well worth the effort. The scenery is mixed—much of the surroundings are industrial, but the river itself and both sides southward are quite attractive. You are also treated to an excellent view of Center City Philadelphia. Expect to encounter a few other people on foot or bicycle. However, large crowds are unlikely.

On the Philadelphia side, the walkway exits at 5th Street. Go left and cross Race Street. 5th Street now takes you past the top historic sites of this city. Pass the Philadelphia U.S. Mint, the world's largest mint, which has been in operation since the inception of the Republic. Pass Christ Church Burial Ground where Benjamin Franklin rests followed by the Liberty Bell pavilion. You then come to Congress Hall, home to

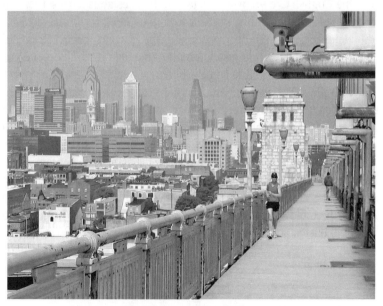

The Benjamin Franklin Bridge Walkway

the House of Representatives and Senate from 1790 to 1800 and where the Bill of Rights was ratified in 1791. After Chestnut Street you come to Independence Hall, where the Declaration of Independence and U.S. Constitution originated. Proceed past Old City Hall and across Walnut Street.

You are now entering the Society Hill neighborhood, famous for its enormous concentration of original 18th and early-19th century architecture. Pick your own way southward through here to South Street, where you should head back eastward towards the river. Around here you can find some excellent pubs, restaurants, and quaint stores. At the corner of South Street and Front Street is our favorite joint, Downey's Irish Pub. It has great food and an impressive décor, including genuine wood paneling, a bar imported from Ireland, and a zillion antiques and memorabilia.

From Downey's, cross Front Street and find the pedestrian bridge across Interstate 95. This brings you to the Independence Seaport Museum. Pass the submarine *USS Becuna* and the cruiser *USS Olympia*—you can tour these if you wish.

Continue north to Penn's Landing. William Penn, an English Quaker, was granted a parcel of land here in 1682, as payment for a debt the English Crown owed his father. Penn established a settlement and named it Philadelphia, derived from the Greek for *brotherly love*. Philadelphia grew rapidly, becoming the second largest English-speaking city in the world just before the American Revolution. Penn's Landing is where Penn first came ashore.

From Penn's Landing you can take the RiverLink Ferry back to Camden. When we were last there, the ferry ran on a 40-minute schedule, so you might want to check a schedule in advance. It is a very pleasant ride.

Back in Camden, you are at the New Jersey State Aquarium (also known as the Adventure Aquarium). Other places of possible interest around here are the Wiggins Park and Amphitheater, Walt Whitman House (three blocks up Mickle Boulevard from the amphitheater), and the Blockbuster-Sony Entertainment Center.

Other Routes

There are many good running and walking routes throughout New Jersey. Here are a few more suggestions of routes close to major centers that happened to come to our attention in our travels of the state.

Hartshorne Woods Park is a 736-acre park in Middletown, Monmouth County, near the mouth of the Navesink River. The main park entrance is at the end of Portland Road, accessed from Route 36. An alternative entrance is off Navesink Road, also accessed from Route 36. There are various loop trails up to six miles long, some being good for running and some being pure hiking trails. There are basic facilities and trail maps at the two entrance points. **Huber Woods Park** is a 357-acre park in Middletown, Monmouth County, accessed from Navesink River Road, off Route 35. There are over seven miles of forested trails, including a trail connection to Hartshorne Woods Park.

The **Henry Hudson Trail** in Monmouth County is a nine-mile long paved rail trail from Lloyd Road, Aberdeen (near Exit 117 of the Garden State parkway), generally following Route 36 to Atlantic Highlands. The eastern terminus is on Route 36, near Avenue D, Atlantic Highlands. There are plans for a twelve-mile extension of this trail from its current western end to Freehold Borough. For more details see www.monmouthcountyparks.com.

The **Loantaka Brook Reservation**, south of Morristown in Morris County, has nearly five miles of paved trails plus additional unpaved trails, all of which are popular with local runners and walkers. The unpaved trails are also occasionally used for horseback riding. The reservation spans Morris, Harding, and Chatham Townships.

Long Branch, Monmouth County, has a boardwalk, about 2.5 miles long, which is popular with runners and walkers. It passes through Pier Village, an attractive and popular seaside center with several restaurants, stores, and other attractions. It also connects to Seven Presidents Ocean Park, Long Branch's main public beach area.

The **Ocean City Boardwalk** (Cape May County) extends a little less than three miles from 1st Street to 23rd Street along the shore in pleasant Ocean City. There is plenty to see and do along the way.

The **Pleasantville-Linwood-Somers Point Bikepath** runs 5.6 miles from Black Horse Pike in Pleasantville to Bethel Road in Somers Point (Atlantic County). This mostly paved trail uses the right-of-way of a trolley car service that once operated between Atlantic City and Ocean City. For more details see www.traillink.com.

The **Saddle River County Park** in Bergen County has a bike and pedestrian path, approximately six miles long, stretching from Ridgewood to Rochelle Park via Glen Rock, Fair Lawn, Paramus, and Saddle Brook. For more details see the Bergen County website www. co.bergen.nj.us.

For more ideas consult the website for New Jersey State Parks at www.state.nj.us/dep/parksandforests or the websites for the various counties, many of which have county parks. For rural trails, consult the website of the New York-New Jersey Trail Conference, Inc. at www. nynjtc.org. Also check out the nearest local running club (see below).

Running Clubs

Atlantic County: Atlantic City RockStar Running (web.mac.com/ acrockstars)
The club mainly coaches young cross-country runners but also trains them for 5K and 10K road races. The club also trains adult runners who are attempting to run the half-marathon or marathon distance. This training is primarily for first or second timers looking to correct issues they had during their first attempt.
Email: rwbuckbee@aol.com

Bergen County: North Jersey Masters Track and Field Club (www. njmasters.com)
North Jersey Masters (NJM), founded in 1976, is based in Ridgewood, Bergen County. The club is dedicated to the improvement of both the recreational and competitive runner from age 18 and older. NJM provides weekly workouts with a professional coach in the spring, summer, and fall, within a supportive and friendly club environment. By running in groups with others of similar speed and ability and by learning training techniques through shared experience, members dramatically improve and reach their potential. The support, wisdom and camaraderie of the club's members has been a successful formula for more than 30 years. NJM organizes the Fred d'Elia Memorial Day Ridgewood Run. There are monthly club meetings with guest speakers, a race of the month, a New York City Marathon bus, and various social activities.
Email: info@njmasters.com

Cumberland County: QuickSilver Track Club of New Jersey (www.qstcnj.org)
This club is based in Vineland, Cumberland County. The club's mission is to train any runner, although its primary athletes are youth. They are mostly athletes from the county but many are from other parts of the state and other states. The club is interested in helping as many as possible to matriculate in the college of their choice, preferably with scholarship support. The athletes regularly compete in spring track programs, summer track, cross country, as well as indoor winter track competition. Athletes compete locally, statewide, and nationally.
Email: qstcnj@aol.com

Essex County: Essex Running Club (www.essexrunning.com)
For a quarter of a century, the Essex Running Club (Essex County) has embraced runners of all types—health-conscious runners (and walkers) seeking to get in shape and stay motivated and fit; competitive runners interested in training, racing, and team events; and adventurous trail runners, ultra-runners, and multi-sport athletes. The club is a source for information, advice, and support; fun and exciting events; camaraderie; and friendship. Monthly club meetings usually feature a speaker and socializing. Group runs range from casual trail runs accommodating all running levels to weekly group training runs to support speed and distance.
Email: Refer to website

Monmouth County: Freehold Area Running Club (www.farcnj. com)
Freehold Area Running Club supports the running community and has promoted running and race walking in central Jersey since 1983. The third largest club in New Jersey, it holds about 25 running events a year. Its activities include weekly group runs (Sundays), group walks (Saturdays) seasonal track sessions (Wednesdays), periodic meetings with guest speakers, newsletters, and social events. The club also supports kids races and awards two-to-five college scholarships each year, depending upon applicants. Many of the club's races are charity events, which typically donate over $25,000 each year to local charities. The club currently has over 400 members. Members include some serious competitors plus many people seeking to just stay in shape.
Email: webmaster@farcnj.com

Monmouth County: Jersey Shore Running Club (www.jsrc.org)
The Jersey Shore Running Club is a local running club with over 2,000 members. It has a diverse and enthusiastic active membership base, with runners of all abilities. Membership is open to all. There are group runs at various locations most days of the week. There are marathon training programs as well as beginner running classes for those interested in getting started. The club stages numerous races throughout the year at all distances from 5Ks to marathons. Events benefit local charitable groups. Anyone is welcome to join in activities posted on the club website, including club runs on Tuesdays, Thursdays, and Sundays.
Email: jsrc@hotmail.com

Monmouth County: New Jersey Road Runners Club (www.njrrc. org)
This club is based in Leonardo, Monmouth County. Its mission is: promoting the sport of running; providing runners of all abilities and goals with the opportunity to train with, learn from, and socialize with those who have similar interests; engaging in community activities and supporting charitable organizations; and educating the public about the health benefits of running for all ages. Members meet for early Sunday morning group runs, regardless of weather. Group runs are generally 6-to-15 miles at various paces. The course can be hilly or flat (along the Henry Hudson Trail), with a mix of paved and gravel surfaces, as well as routes through Huber Woods and Hartshorne Woods on rough dirt trails. The club hosts several races in Monmouth County.
Email: info@njrrc.org

Morris County: Amazing Feet Running Club (www.amazingfeetrc. com)
This club welcomes runners of all levels from Morris, Union, and Somerset Counties. The group has regular training runs of 3-to-20 miles, with all paces welcome. There are Saturday morning runs at Loantaka Brook Reservation, South Street entrance, in Morris County. On Sundays there are various country runs, followed by breakfast.
Email: rob@brigham-rago.com or chickrun@patmedia.net

Morris County: Morris County Striders (www.morriscountystriders. com)
The Morris County Striders are a mix of open and masters runners, primarily long distance roads and cross-country with some track.

Group runs take place several days of the week in various locations. Skill levels range from beginner to experienced competitive local elite. The club hosts a summer cross country series in Boonton Township and a local road race in June in Roxbury Township. Club members have a close bond and enjoy post race get-togethers as well as club-organized social events throughout the year.
Email: pjfales@hotmail.com

Morris County: The Original Geezers (No website)
This Randolph-based club is semi-competitive and highly social. Members are mostly 45 and over males, but others of all ages and gender are welcome. There are Saturday or Sunday runs and team races. The club assists in a local 5K held every October.
Email: plee@us.fujitsu.com

Morris County: Rose City Runners (www.rosecityrunners.com)
This club, based in Madison, Morris County, targets anyone interested in running for fitness or competition. The club has members of all ages from 20s to 80s. Members meet every Saturday morning at Loantaka Park in Morris Township, for a group run followed by breakfast. There are typically 30 or more runners of varying speeds. Club member spouses can walk and then join the runners at breakfast. The club hosts several races, numerous social events, and some non-running trips away. The club also has a USATF racing team.
Email: Refer to website

Passaic County: Clifton Roadrunners Club
(www.cliftonroadrunners.com)
This club serves mid-to-northern New Jersey. Its mission is to provide runners of all ages and all abilities, from the recreational to the competitive runner, a club where they can share the miles with runners of similar pace and interest. Members run distances from track to marathons. Their times are from 17 to 45 minutes for a 5K and 3 to 6 hours for a marathon. The youngest member is four (one-mile distance) and the oldest running member is 68. There are weekly and weekend group runs at Brookdale Park (two-mile loop) or Saddle Brook Park (eight-mile loop). The club hosts winter runs, track workouts, marathon training, a 50-mile one-day relay, car-pooling to Central Park races, and social events.
Email: bobbaloonie@comcast.net

Somerset County: The Sudden Impact Track Club (www. suddenimpact-track.org)
This Somerset-based club is for youth athletes. Its purpose is to provide a no-nonsense environment for those athletes who are serious about competitive running.
Email: info@suddenimpact-track.org

Special Olympics New Jersey (www.sonj.org)
This organization holds various fundraising activities around the state to benefit more than 17,000 athletes of Special Olympics New Jersey. Events include the Lincoln Tunnel Challenge 5K Fun Run/Walk in April, the Jersey Shore Running Club's Walk for Special Olympics New Jersey in April, and the Lawrence Loop Run/Walk in October in Lawrenceville, NJ.
Email: ljs@sonj.org

Union County: Central Jersey Road Runners Club (www.cjrrc. org)
Central Jersey Road Runners Club (CJRRC) is dedicated to promoting running and racing to people of all ages, encouraging camaraderie among all runners, and educating people about how to run safely and smartly. CJRRC has members ranging in age from teens to 80s; some run a few miles a week, some ultra distances. All abilities are welcome and supported. Some runners are highly competitive and others run for recreation and good health. The club holds regular meetings in Cranford, featuring guest speakers on topics of interest to runners. It sponsors three races annually, offers running classes for beginning and experienced runners at two New Jersey locations, and has group social events including an annual picnic at Monmouth Racetrack.
Email: Refer to website

The Shore Athletic Club of New Jersey (www.shoreac.org)
The Shore Athletic Club fields "varsity" and local men's and women's teams competing in every event within the track and field sport, and on every level, youth to juniors to "open" to Sub-Masters and Masters. There are over 500 members. Most but not all live in New Jersey. The club also puts on at least 75 events for all comers. The club caps each year with a January awards banquet. The work gets done through the team efforts of a group of volunteers and good friends.
Email: Refer to website

12

Conclusion

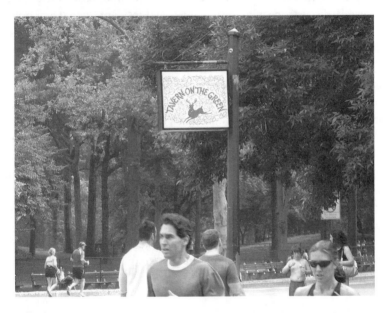

Our last photo shows the end point of the New York City Marathon, by Tavern on the Green in Central Park, on a typical summer day. New York City and its surrounds provide an outstanding opportunity for on-foot exercise, whether that be running, jogging, or walking. There are many excellent trails close to where most of us live or stay, and many community activities, such as running clubs, to help get us all outdoors more.

Our main objective in this book has been to point you to some of the best places to exercise, with the hope that you will spend more time outdoors, becoming fitter, faster, and (if applicable to you) more successful in your on-foot competition.

Regardless of your age, fitness level, special limitations, and speed, you can very likely extend your life and improve your quality of life by spending more time outdoors on foot. It is never too late to start exercising more.

Documenting the best on-foot exercise routes around New York City plus the major centers of New York State and New Jersey is no easy task. It is not even a feasible task, since there are so many great places to run or walk in this part of the world. What we have done is try to capture the very best routes we could find, based on general research, discussions with local athletes and residents, and many miles of personal on-foot slogging (much of it unfruitful, but still not a loss since it helped keep us fit).

We know many of you will have a favorite route that is not included in this book. Please do not be shy in contacting us (through the www.funonfoot.com website) with your thoughts, so we can consider including your ideas in future revisions of this book.

We also urge you to find and work with your own local running club, for encouragement, camaraderie, and support. There are so many excellent clubs in the New York and New Jersey region there was no way we could mention them all. We welcome all approaches from running clubs for inclusion on our website or future revisions of this book.

Best wishes in your endeavors towards keeping fit and lengthening your lives. Running and walking in and around New York can really be fun!

Index

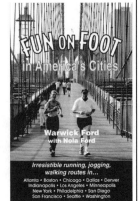

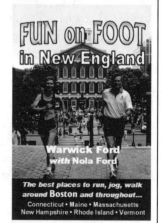

About the Authors

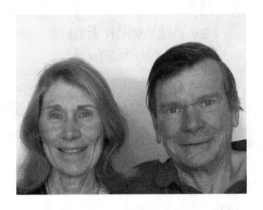

Warwick Ford and Nola Ford are Australian-raised Canadian-Americans with a passion for running, skiing, and other outdoor activities. They have lived in the U.S.A. since 1996, mainly based in Massachusetts but spending significant time in New York throughout. They run regularly in community races in New York and elsewhere, with Warwick racing up to the half-marathon distance. They love exploring new territory on foot, while maintaining fitness at the same time. Their main mission currently is to help others keep fit by documenting the results of these on-foot explorations. Warwick's educational qualifications include a Ph. D. from the University of Toronto. In his earlier career, he authored technical books including *Computer Communications Security* and *Secure Electronic Commerce*.

By the Same Authors:
Fun on Foot in America's Cities
Fun on Foot in New England